I SURVIVED CANCER

But Never Won
The Tour de France

I SURVIVED CANCER

But Never Won
The Tour de France

Jim Chastain

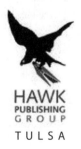

HAWK
PUBLISHING
GROUP

TULSA

LIBRARY OF CONGRESS CATALOG IN PUBLICATION DATA

I Survived Cancer but Never Won the Tour de France /Jim Chastain

[1. Jim Chastain - Non-Fiction-United States.]

Cover Design by Müllerhaus Publishing Arts, Inc. | mhpubarts.com

ISBN 1-930709-60-9
Library of Congress Control Number: 2006929278

Published in the United States by HAWK Publishing Group.

HAWK Publishing Group
7107 South Yale Avenue #345
Tulsa, OK 74136
918-492-3677
HawkPub.com
HeartlandAuthors.com

HAWK and colophon are trademarks belonging to the HAWK
Publishing Group. Printed in the United States of America.
9 8 7 6 5 4 3 2 1

For LeAnn, Maddye, and Ford,
who were with me through it all.

Contents

Introduction

The title of this book is presumptuous, I'll admit, for as I began writing this book at the beginning of 2003, I didn't really know if I would survive cancer. Indeed, there continues to be speculation on this subject, and the stakes are now higher than ever.

Such is the world of the "cancer survivor." You're never quite sure if the disease is really gone or what future problems you'll face as a result of your efforts fighting it off.

I was first diagnosed with malignant fibrous hystiocytoma, a type of soft tissue sarcoma, in August of 2001, several months after discovering a tiny lump in the triceps muscle of my right arm and having it biopsied. I was then a 37-year-old lawyer for the State of Oklahoma with a wife and two kids. And boy was I scared.

I had surgery at M.D. Anderson Cancer Center in Houston the following month and then six weeks of "radiation therapy" (an oxymoron if ever there was one) in Oklahoma City. The worst of it seemed to be behind me. The doctors gave me a 90% chance of never seeing the cancer again.

But nearly a year to the day after my original diagnosis, another lump appeared in virtually the same spot. In October of 2002, doctors confirmed that cancer had returned, meaning it had never really been gone in the first place. Surgery (my third) followed sixteen days later. After that, I had a painful radiation procedure that required me to be quarantined in an isolated room at M.D. Anderson for several days.

Shortly thereafter, I began writing this book. It was therapeutic. Writing about my experiences helped to relieve some of the pressure. Managing cancer is mostly about managing stress. And for me, writing was the answer.

You see, during the worst days, those initial days when everything seemed so dark and confusing and scary, I'd started writing monthly updates to friends and family to let them know how things were progressing with my health. This kept those close to me informed and at the same time prevented me from having to tell the same traumatic news over and over again. In other words, a win-win situation.

The updates were a surprising hit. My family, friends, and coworkers actually looked forward to reading them—at least that's what they said. People I didn't know from places I'd never heard of would send e-mails telling me how much they'd enjoyed reading my update that so-and-so had forwarded.

Over time, people I respected began encouraging me to turn my updates into a book. Although I wasn't sure the updates were book material, I decided to follow their advice, up to a point. The book would cover only the most surreal moments, events that were particularly funny, frightening, or sad. In other words, the moments that were most interesting, from a human point of view. Writing about my experiences seemed crucial for some reason, regardless of whether or not the material was ever published.

I'd completed a first draft of the book by the end of August, 2003. But my cancer journey was far from over. In November of that year, doctors discovered the cancer had returned once again. This time I had three tumors in my arm, not one. The biggest tumor was near my armpit, and one trustworthy doctor described it as "ominous."

And so, after consulting with a team of cancer experts, I had my entire triceps muscle removed in a difficult surgery (my fourth) in December of 2003. This left my arm in a permanently handicapped condition. But I could still write. I added two more chapters in January of 2004 and called it a book.

I have "survived" cancer...for two and a half years anyway. But that doesn't mean the danger is over. The cancer has recurred twice. My arm is mangled and forever flawed. I am still under constant medical surveillance, and there continues to be great concern about my health. We no longer talk about odds and probabilities; with me, such talk would be pure guesswork. We talk about keeping hope, having good days, and making time count.

And so, I don't really know if I'll survive cancer. That is part of the dilemma, part of the journey, part of the learning process, and part of the pain. But in choosing a title for my book, it seemed a bit of optimism was needed. For I doubt anyone would care to read a book called, *I May Soon Die of Cancer, and the Tour de France Isn't on my Radar Screen.*

So what, you may ask, is this book all about? Perhaps it is easier to tell you what it's not. It's not a celebrity's cancer book, for in the grand scheme of things, I'm pretty much a nobody—just a lawyer who works at an appellate court and writes poetry and newspaper articles on the side. It's not a "miracle cure" book, for I'm no shaman. I have no magic words or potions that will fix you, or make cancer go away. It's not a "how-to" book with in-depth details about a particular kind of cancer. There are plenty of those around, written by people who know a lot more about the mechanics and science of cancer than I do. I have little to say about the stages of grief, the best cancer centers for your money, or the latest treatments, simply because I'm not an expert on such things. This is more of a tour than a battle plan.

From the outset, I wanted to write something different. Something that addresses the strange paradoxes of cancer, what I call the *wow moments.* A funny, yet brutally honest look at a young family trying to survive in crisis mode. A book that will surely make you laugh, but isn't afraid to make you cry.

This book is about telling stories, real stories that made me pause and say, "Can you believe that really happened?" Some would call it a memoir, but it's more like a series of vivid snapshots of the highest highs, lowest lows, and weirdest weirds.

One of my biggest goals was to write a book that cancer patients and their families could relate to, but one that could also be enjoyed by those without any connection to cancer at all. In other words, I wanted to write the type of book I was looking for when I was first diagnosed with cancer, but never found. In attempting to fulfill that mission, I focused my writing on five practical needs that cancer patients typically experience: the need to laugh; the need to be real; the need to know (that is, to receive valuable insider information on what cancer is like); the need to be known; and the need to find hope.

This book examines each of these needs in a series of seventeen "cancer stories" from my life during the past three years. The simple intent is to record the strange, fascinating, and often surreal things that have happened. At the end, I hope you will be shaking your head and saying, "Isn't life crazy?"

For you see, to put it in Lance Armstrong terminology, "it's not about the tumor." If anything, this book is about that elusive search for meaning in life. Cancer is the catalyst in this book, but it's not the main character. We are.

And now for a little c.y.a.

Writing about one's life experiences is difficult, because the writer risks relationships in relating what has been seen and suffered through. This is probably why many writers turn to fiction, which is so often nonfiction artfully disguised.

Ultimately, the writer must decide whether or not to (1) tell a story exactly as he or she remembers it in order to get to the underlying truth, or (2) soften the blow, in order to preserve relationships and keep his or her house from getting egged. The best writers stick with option one. The ones who never get published usually opt for option two. Because this is a memoir, with very little room for poetic license, I tried to stick with option one. Even so, I'm trying to be both as real and as kind as I can.

My sincerest apologies go out to anyone who remembers events differently or who feels slighted by my recollections in any way. Even though you're wrong, I recognize your right to be wrong. This is, after all, a free country.

But seriously, my intention is to give an accurate account, not to take potshots at anyone. I tell it like it is, realizing all the while people aren't perfect and in most circumstances are just trying to do the best they can.

And finally, let me say this, for the record: Lance Armstrong is an incredible athlete who deserves all the praise, accolades, and book deals he can get. I hope to meet him someday, perhaps when I'm signing his copy of my book.

I'm kidding, of course. For if anything is abundantly clear, it's that I'm no Lance Armstrong. But hopefully my cancer experiences are not any less relevant simply because I hate exercise.

March, 2004.

CRAZY

let's stay up all night
ignoring this crazy world
laughing while we can

1

Nothing

We have nothing to fear, but fear itself.
— paraphrased from FDR's first inaugural address

Nothing gold can stay.
— from *Nothing Gold Can Stay,* by Robert Frost

My old life ended and a new one began with a short snow cone trip in May of 2001.

That day, some friends stopped by our house to see if the Chastain family (Jim, LeAnn, Madison, and Ford) wanted to go out for a snow cone. Norman, Oklahoma has a great snow cone place, so it didn't take much convincing to get us to join them.

Besides, we're sugar freaks. We do this sort of thing all the time.

We loaded into our junky old van (now retired, thankfully), an embarrassing vehicle with just enough room to hold six sugar-starved people in need of a quick fix. The kids jumped in the back, our friend Gina sat in the middle with her son Andrew, and LeAnn took her normal spot in the front passenger seat. I drove, because, well, that's what I do.

We set forth on a short jaunt across town, talking, laughing, and listening to the radio, the typical sort of things people do. Life, as they say, was good.

But how quickly things can change. Perhaps a mile or so before we reached our destination, I felt an itch near my right elbow. I reached over and scratched it; after all, that's what one does with an itch. "Ah-hhh," I thought, as I contemplated what flavor of snow cone I would soon be devouring.

But as I finished scratching, my hand dragged across the underside of my upper right arm. And there it came to an abrupt stop at what would prove to be a crossroad.

What is that? I wondered.

It was a whelp or knot or...something. Tiny, yes, but noticeable all the same. Had I been bitten by a bug? I didn't think so. There were no visible bite marks on my skin. Plus, it didn't really feel like a bite; it was actually *below* the skin. In fact, the bump seemed to be on the arm muscle, whatever that's called. (The triceps muscle, for those of you keeping score.)

Meanwhile, the van conversation continued. Andrew was doing this and that. Madison's swimming was going well. Ford was probably going to play baseball this year. Gina had just finished reading a good book.

But I wasn't participating in the conversation. For me, time was standing still. In some sense, I had left the van entirely. I was off in some distant lonely place, trying my best to explain away a tiny little lump.

What in the world is it?

There were hundreds of possibilities. Perhaps I'd bumped my arm against something and caused inflammation. I'd been drinking a lot of coffee—maybe it was some sort of caffeine buildup. Or maybe it was a fatty deposit. Gross yes, but not dangerous to anything but pride.

Perhaps it was a rogue piece of tissue that had broken off and decided to go on a journey. Maybe it was an ingrown hair or an internal pimple, if there was such a thing.

Surely it was nothing to worry about.

But a voice deep inside me—the internal alarm clock that occasionally awakens one's soul from a peaceful slumber—had its own theory: This was a tumor. In fact, the alarm clock had a more specific opinion than that, but I tried my best to ignore such prognostications. *Don't even go there,* I told myself.

We reached our destination and piled out of the van. As family and friends began walking to the snow cone stand, I pulled my wife aside for a panicky chat.

"Hey, feel this place right here," I said. "There's something on my arm."

LeAnn did what I asked in a quick, preoccupied way. I guided her to the spot and moved her fingers across it.

"Huh," she said, with a half curious, half disinterested tone, like one might use upon seeing a new McDonalds in your hometown.

"Can you feel it?" I asked.

"Yeah. Did you hit your arm or something?"

"I don't think so," I answered, reviewing the last two weeks of my life in a few anxious seconds. I looked deeply into her eyes, waiting for some much-deserved reassurance.

"Well..." she said. "I'm sure it's nothing." Then she turned and joined the others.

Nothing. That was her diagnosis.

I'm not really sure what I had expected her to do. Give me an in depth medical opinion? Of course not. Burst out crying? Not hardly. Rush me to a hospital? It was way too early for anything like that.

It's not like the sky was falling, Chicken Little. Not yet anyway.

LeAnn had simply reached the same conclusion many others after her would reach: the lump was nothing. It was just some tightness or swelling in my arm, and there was absolutely no reason to think otherwise. After all, I was thirty-seven years old. The odds were clearly in my favor.

Try as I might, though, I was unable to reach the same conclusion. This was not nothing. It was something. The question was whether it was a good something or a bad something. And that was a pretty unsettling question to leave hanging out there, unanswered.

So the next day, I phoned my doctor. I call him my doctor, but that's kind of a stretch. More precisely, he's a doctor who had seen me twice for something extremely embarrassing. Then, I'd had no choice but to go see him. This time the visit was purely discretionary.

In hindsight, my decision to call a doctor was not only unlikely, it was miraculous. I hadn't been to a doctor's office in years. My history with annual checkups was unimpressive. The only time I went to the doctor was when surgery was required.

But as luck would have it, my doctor was gone for the day. This was bad timing, not only because of my sporadic decision to go there, but also because my wife and I were leaving for vacation the next week. I needed to know what, if anything, was wrong with me as soon as possible.

Hmmm...what to do.

I considered waiting until after we'd returned from vacation to have the "nothing" examined. After all, it was my normal practice to procrastinate to a fault. Instead, I scheduled an appointment with another doctor. I was restless and in need of some answers.

This new doctor was a big man, more like a football player than a doctor. I don't remember his name, but he would become one of several people who helped save my life.

The doctor felt my arm. He paused. He shifted. He scratched his chin. He asked me some doctor-type questions. When did I first notice this? Had I recently hit my arm on something? Did I have a problem with ingrown hairs or internal pimples?

"It's probably nothing," he said. "But...I think we should do an ultrasound, just to be safe. No, let's make that an MRI."

An MRI? I sort of knew what an MRI was, but only vaguely. It had something to do with a tube, didn't it? To be honest, at that particular moment, I was probably more concerned about how much an MRI would cost than I was about the procedure itself. Nevertheless, the MRI chamber would soon become a regular part of this roller coaster I would continuously ride for months upon months.

I had the MRI the next day and was sent home to await the results.

Ah, waiting for test results—one of life's most excruciating disciplines.

Nothing can make a grown man feel more helpless and exasperated than the time spent waiting impatiently for a phone call about test results. It didn't help that I had unresolved scheduling issues. LeAnn and I were now one week away from vacation—a cruise with my parents, sisters, and my sisters' husbands. Would I be going on a cruise ship or an operating table? From surgery to suntan lotion, there was a lot at stake.

But doctors and lab techs tend to see things differently. They don't get overly concerned about such trivialities as pre-purchased vacation packages and unbearable waiting-for-the-results stress. Time is of the essence for almost everyone they see, and so they treat everyone equally slow.

Insofar as test results are concerned, you generally don't get a quick answer unless you know someone on the inside. I didn't. And if you think you're going to get preferential treatment because you're going on a cruise, you can forget about it. That sort of reason can delay your test results by another two days!

The logic seems to go like this—everyone's in the same boat here, so just sit back, relax, and be patient. (Indeed, that's why we're called "patients.")

So I waited. And I waited. And I waited some more.

One day passed and then another. By the end of day three, we still had no news about the nothing.

Meanwhile, the lengthy delay had tripled my capacity for dreaming up Oliver Stone-like conspiracy theories. I began to imagine the radiologist's thought processes as he considered my scans. He surely said something like, "I guess I could write up that report tonight and get it to Mr. Chastain, who seems to be freaking out a bit and has a trip planned. But he needs to learn right now that this isn't about him."

Anyway, with my nerves shot, my good health on the line, and a cruise at stake, I was growing increasingly restless. At some point, I was unable to wait any longer. So I went into lawyer mode, using my legal experience to bypass the system and obtain some insider information.

After making several phone calls and possibly even hiding my identity here and there, I was able to obtain the phone number of the radiologist who would be reading my MRI and reporting his conclusions. I called his office, after hours, hoping to catch him off guard.

I did.

"Oh, yes. Mr. Chastine..."

"It's Chastain."

"Uh-huh. I was just looking at your MRI. Let's see, it's here somewhere." (I seem to remember the sound of papers rattling, a drink being poured over ice, and a disconcerting giggle in the background, although this may be due to my overactive imagination.) "I've dictated the report, but it won't be typed until tomorrow."

"Oh," I said painfully, as I calculated another eight hours of continuous trips to the bathroom while waiting. "It's just that we've got this trip planned, and everyone's waiting to hear if we're going to get to go," I said.

Notice I didn't say cruise. I'd quickly learned that cruise is a buzzword for spoiled rich kid, which I'm not, unless you live on some continent other than North America, Europe, and possibly Australia. If I had used the word cruise, I would then be obliged to tell him the rest of the pathetic story, that this was my first cruise and my parents were paying for it, even though I was thirty-seven years old.

The additional information wouldn't completely remove spoiled rich kid from the mix, but it would suggest that, if I am rich, it's not my fault. "Could you bend the rules just this once?" I asked, cutting to the chase.

"Well, I'm not supposed to..." he replied. I imagined his darting eyes looking around the room for the hospital watchdogs who would surely fire him if he was caught revealing test results too soon, i.e., before my pulse had risen to a dangerously high level.

"But if you won't tell anyone..." he said.

"Oh, I won't," I lied.

"Listen, Mr. Chastine. Everything is just fine," he lied back. "There is like a 99.9 percent chance that this is absolutely nothing."

Nothing? Did I hear that right?

The lump really was nothing!

A huge burst of air exploded from me, like a bear's fart following a salmon binge. Not only was this something nothing, it was "absolutely" nothing, which surely meant something very close to a sure thing. My relief was greater than I can put into words.

"It's nodular fasciitis, which is a benign growth. I mean, there's always that remote other possibility, but I wouldn't get worked up about it. I'll have to do some CYA in the report, of course, and list some other possibilities. And you may want to get it biopsied somewhere down the road, just to be sure, but I'm not worried about it."

He wasn't worried about it. But why should he be? After all, to this unseen man, whomever he was, I was just a name on a page, a shadowy appendage on an MRI photograph, Mr. Chastine. True, I was also now a voice, but without a face and some background details, I was about as real as plastic surgery.

But still, he said it was a nodule. That was surely very common. I was fine. I would live!

I passed this joyous news on to my wife, kids, friends, parents, sisters, boss, coworkers, and a few total strangers, just for good measure. And one by one, most of them would tell me, "I knew it was nothing." One of the strangers even burst out crying.

A doctor called the next day to report the same glorious news, not knowing I had already spoken to the radiologist and been faxed a copy of the report. "It's nothing," he reported. "Just a strained muscle."

"No it's not." I said. "It's nodular fasciitis."

"You have the report?" he said. "How did...?"

"I called the radiologist and had him fax it to me."

"Oh," he said. (Muffled sound of sharp talking to some assistant type here.) "Well, nodular fasciitis...That's just a fancy schmancy way of saying tendonitis. A trauma to the arm."

"It is?" I asked.

"Yes," he said, unconvincingly. "The bottom line is it's nothing. So go on your cruise, relax, and enjoy yourself, okay? Forget about it."

"What about when I get back? Should I come in for a biopsy? The report says I might want to have one, just to be sure."

"Well sure, you can have it biopsied in a couple of months, if you want. But for now, I'd just watch it."

That was the advice. Just watch it. Statistically speaking, I had nothing to worry about.

This would become a bothersome pattern in my life. In the coming months, I would be told over and over again that this lump in my arm (or the ones that followed) was nothing—nothing to be concerned with anyway. Forget about it. Eat, drink, and be merry; it's tomorrow that you may die.

I hung up the phone and smiled. This was nothing. Really nothing.

But my alarm clock, which had heard the word "biopsy," still said otherwise. And it continued to do so, until I ultimately learned the alarm clock had been right from the very beginning.

For what it's worth, when it comes to making decisions about one's health, you simply can't pass the buck to someone else. Regardless of the stress involved, nobody is more in tune with your own body than you. Not your doctor, your radiologist, or your full time caregiver. Not your spouse, your family members, or your best friend. Everything ultimately depends on what *you* decide to do.

No matter what you may think, doctors are not all-seeing or all-knowing. They are humans, after all, and most of them are way too busy. At times, the best information doctors may have is some statistical probabilities. And so, when they say just wait and watch it, it will be up to you to calculate in the catastrophe that awaits if they're wrong.

To wait might fall in line with the odds, but, from a personal point-of-view, the risk of waiting could be sky high.

You are the one with the alarm clock. You have to make that life-saving call.

I didn't listen to the probabilities. I had the biopsy done, after the cruise anyway, and learned the nothing was a very serious something.

And that, my friends, made quite a difference.

NEVER, NEVER LAND

I once thought my thirty-six year old uncle
was ancient or at least very advanced in years.
Now I long to be thirty-six again
and to stay there forever. Or, even better,

to age backwards—growing younger each year,
wrinkles disappearing, hair reappearing,
more spring in my step, and a less jaded point
of view, until one day I'm a kid once more,

like those old people in *The Twilight Zone*,
running giddy around the playground,
kicking the can without a care in the world.
At forty, there are plenty of concerns.

Trouble howls out in the night, surrounds
you like a pack of ravenous wolves.
Oh, to be young again! Bring on
the broken hearts, bad haircuts, braces,

puberty, acne, peer pressure, proms,
arch-enemies, homework, and first love.
I'll behave myself better this time.
Peter Pan had it right, I think.

2

Regarding Lance Armstrong

My daughter Madison had an upcoming swim meet in Bartlesville, Oklahoma—my former hometown. Since Bartlesville was a three-hour drive from our current home, my family made plans for a weekend getaway.

The meet would be held in the very same pool where I once learned to swim (but never quite graduated from swimming classes). We would be staying with my parents, who still live in Bartlesville.

These are fun times for us—these trips home—because we get to relax, read, let the kids run wild, and eat like there's no tomorrow. Sometimes, LeAnn and I even leave the kids with my parents and sneak away for coffee or a movie.

Of course, these trips home aren't completely stress free. There's a definite price to pay. That is, unless I just happen to be in the mood to listen to my parents talk about church for the greater part of two days.

My parents talk incessantly about church, i.e., *their* church. Things are going quite well there apparently, and they love to drive that point home. It's like a broken record—Mom and Dad's personalized version of *Stairway to Heaven*. So and so just joined the church. Remodeling is coming in ahead of schedule. Dad is on this or that committee. The pastor's sermon was a real keeper.

Yikes!

My parents just don't seem to get it. Even when I tell them upfront, "I don't want to talk about church," they keep right on going. They say something like, "Why not? Is there something wrong at your church? Because at our church..."

Oh well. What can you do?

Anyway, I called Mom to let her know when we would arrive for the big swim meet. This is critical information, because my parents plan their lives around meals. Literally. My sisters and I are expected to give at least two days notice of our estimated time of arrival so that all the food arrangements can be settled. After that, the various meals and, more importantly, the time for those meals are set in stone.

Nothing else goes on the schedule of events until all meals are in place. Nothing!

Consequently, my parents—and by my parents, I mean my Dad—tend to get irritated when I'm not sure when my family will arrive. And God help us if I tell them we'll be there for dinner, but then get caught in traffic along the way.

I can see my father now, standing in front of the window, waiting for the Prodigal to return. "Where is that boy? It's time to eat! He's going to make me late for church."

Anyway, I told my mom our plans, and she relayed all the pertinent details to my father as he took notes. Why notes? So he could type them into his computer and print out a helpful agenda:

6:10 p.m. Serve dinner: Mexican chicken, salad, rolls, chocolate shortcake, and dip for Jimmy.

6:11 p.m. Talk about church.

Mom scanned her agenda and let me know what was on the weekend's menu. She then gave me her week's highlights, i.e., how many times she'd been to church, where they'd eaten, and what new vacation she and Dad were planning.

But then she added something different. Something sinister and, quite frankly, alarming.

"Oh, by the way, *your* grandmother wants to see you."

"She does?" I said, followed by a long, suspicious pause. "Why?"

Truth be known, I was pretty sure I knew why Grandma wanted to see me. But I wasn't going to let on just yet. I wanted to make Mom squirm a little.

You see, I was almost certain this was going to be the obligatory cancer call. Grandma was simply following protocol. I'd recently been diagnosed with a rare form of cancer, and Grandma was now expected to make face-to-face contact "just in case."

I figured Mom was behind it, for this had her name written all over it. She'd probably suggested, in the way moms do, that Grandma spend some quality time with me, RIGHT NOW! Most likely the conversation went something like this: "He's such a nice boy, you know. You should call him. Or better yet, come see him." It was either that guilt trip or Grandma had, for the first time that I can remember, decided to come see me all on her own.

Whatever the case, I wanted Mom to admit the truth: that, on some level, this was about expectations and appearances. But before we could get there, she would have to tap dance.

"Oh...she just wants to see you." Mom said. "She's getting older, you know, and she wants to get to know you better. She doesn't really know you all that well, and she wants to."

"Well, why now?" I asked in a sarcastic tone. "I'm thirty-eight years old. Why am I so interesting now?"

To explain why my grandmother and I are virtual strangers would take more space than we have here. Suffice it to say there had been a nasty divorce a long time ago, and as a result my mom was not raised by her mother, but by her grandmother. For me, this situation led to less grand-motherly contact than one might typically expect. In fact, I had long since come to think of Grandma as something akin to a great aunt.

"I guess she hears me talking about you all the time, and, since you're never around for Christmas, she doesn't have the chance to see for herself what a wonderful guy you are," Mom replied.

Touché. Mom knows how to play the game, juxtaposing the adjective wonderful against my unforgivable actions with respect to Christmas.

Yes, this was my passive-aggressive mom in rare form, laying on another guilt trip in order to keep me off the trail. Now we were suddenly on the topic of Christmas, how I had decided a few years back to forego the family tradition of driving three and a half hours on Christmas morning to see a lot of relatives I barely know. Mom had disagreed with that decision, and she liked to remind me of that fact periodically. It seems that every year I'm the only one in the extended family, excluding one jailbird cousin, who doesn't make it back for the holiday celebration.

I needed to steer her back to the real issue at hand: an out-of-the blue meeting with Grandma.

"So, it's just me she wants to see?" I asked. "She didn't say anything about my kids or LeAnn?" *Take that!* I'd avoided the whole Christmas issue by asking a question of my own. The chess match continued, and it was Mom's move.

"Well sure, she wants to see them too, of course she does. But she's particularly interested in seeing you," she explained.

"Huh...Well, she should come to Norman then, if she wants to see me. We're always home."

"I'm not talking about that," she replied.

"What *are* you talking about?" I asked.

"Well," Mom said. "I think your grandmother's going to stop by this weekend...when you're in town."

And so it began.

This was just like my mother. The meeting with Grandma had already been placed on the agenda. Mom was just giving me the heads-up.

Now, don't get me wrong. It's not that I dislike my Grandma or anything. Let's make that fact perfectly clear. We've never had any problems at all. She seems just as nice as the next great aunt.

It's just I don't know her that well. I mean, I know she's friendly, has four nice kids, attends a charismatic church, and has a new set of dentures. But that's about all I know.

Plus, I'm not really good at these forced conversations. That's where my wife shines. I, however, tend to freeze in uncomfortable situations. I stutter on my words, throwing in "uhs" and "you knows," as if I'd never gone to college. Small talk just isn't my thing, especially when it's really not small talk at all, but something with a greater purpose in mind.

Be that as it may, the meeting with Grandma was already on the agenda, at 12:48 p.m., just before pot roast and a brief discussion about the church's new carpet.

We arrived in Bartlesville a few days later. Madison completed her morning swims, and then we drove to Mom and Dad's house for lunch. Dad clocked me in, and Mom pointed me toward the den, where Grandma was waiting.

I entered the room, said hi, and gave her the obligatory hug. Then I headed for the back bedroom to collect my thoughts.

How long would it take before we got to the cancer part? Would we just hem and haw around the subject? Would she try to lay hands on me or anoint me with oil? It was hard to know how this was going to play out.

After ten minutes, when I hadn't reappeared, LeAnn came to the rescue. She urged me to go in and get it over with, in the way wives do. (Something like, "Get in there, you big chicken!")

I set forth like a man condemned.

Grandma sat on the sofa, looking a bit uncomfortable as I entered the room. I'm sure this was no picnic for her either. I mean, what was she supposed to say to her grandson who had been diagnosed with cancer?

Grandma cleared her throat and shifted about nervously. She seemed incapable of looking me straight in the eye, which was not unusual in those days. Cancer and direct eye contact seemed to be mutually exclusive.

I took a seat in a chair some fifteen feet or so away from her. This was surely not the best distance in the world to have meaningful conversation or suddenly form a lasting relationship. But the distance between us made me feel a little more relaxed.

"So how are you doing, Jimmy Lee?" she asked, using my elementary school nickname.

Asking someone how they are doing is a pretty safe conversation starter, under normal circumstances, but a loaded gun when you pose it to one who has been struggling with cancer. Armed with a question like that, I could, if I so desired, bring my grandmother to her arthritic knees. I could say something like, "Awesome! Cancer's been a total blast!"

But one cannot say such things to one's grandmother, at least not in a civilized world. I had to answer the question honestly and somehow suppress my tendencies toward sarcasm.

"Oh, I'm doing okay, I guess. Right now, anyway...knock on wood."

A little lame, yes, but that was the best I could come up with on the spur of the moment.

I think the idea of knocking on wood probably sounded too mystical, too Tom Cruise, for poor Grandma. She was quiet for a moment, possibly confused, unsure where to go next. This conversation was going to be a bit tricky, for her own grandson had just suggested he was relying on hocus-pocus superstitions for healing, instead of God.

The time was ripe for a segue.

"Yes...So, have you been following the Tour de France?" she asked with a poker face.

The Tour de France? Was she kidding?

Anyone who's ever had cancer can spot this conversation a mile away. The Tour de France means Lance Armstrong. Lance Armstrong means young man with cancer. Young man with cancer who *survived*. Young man with cancer who survived and beat the odds and then went on to win the grueling Tour de France, supposedly the world's toughest race, multiple times.

Armstrong's bestselling book, *It's Not About the Bike*, taunted me every time I went to the bookstore. For a person still trying to defeat cancer (and a non-celebrity at that), these "you can conquer the world" books can be...intimidating. There was Lance smiling at the top of the mountain, while I hadn't even made it to base camp.

Be that as it may, Lance Armstrong was going to be Grandma's pathway to meaningful conversation, and I had no choice but to ride along.

"The Tour de France?" I asked, as if puzzled. "No, not really. I don't really follow it. I mean, except what I read in the headlines."

On the list of sports I might watch on television, bicycling would rank pretty far down there, somewhere after table tennis, but before bowling, car racing, and ice skating (unless Nancy Kerrigan and Tonya Harding went at it again).

"That American is winning it. I can't remember his name, but he's won it before." She was acting as though I'd had my head buried in the sand for the last several years. No, I don't "follow" the Tour de France, but I am a guy. I still watch Sports Center at least twice a week.

"Yes, Lance Armstrong. He's...impressive," I offered.

"He sure is," she observed.

Here, there was an excruciatingly long pause.

"You know...he had cancer."

There. She'd said it. Now we could both breathe a little easier.

"Yes. I heard that," I said, in a slower, respectful way, as if honoring a fallen war hero.

"And he survived. Just look at him now, winning that bike race and all. That can't be easy," Grandma observed.

"He's pretty...impressive," I offered, again.

"Yes. And then there's that baseball player," she said, switching gears.

Baseball? Where was she going with that? Darryl Strawberry perhaps? No. He had survived cancer, but with all his past drug problems Grandma would hardly be singing his praises.

Wait a minute. Surely she wasn't going there.

"Dave Dravecky?" I asked, connecting the dots.

"Yes! He had cancer in his arm too. Of course things didn't work out so well for him..." She shook her head, out of respect for the now armless pitcher.

"Yes..." I said, suddenly unable to think clearly.

Although Dravecky is surely a hero and a truly courageous man, he was still not someone I liked to think about a lot during my cancer struggles, for obvious arm-related reasons. Dravecky was a great role model, but his predicament was exactly what I was hoping to avoid.

What a great pep talk this had turned out to be!

I really can't remember where the conversation went from there. I think Grandma presented her spiritual take on things, throwing out some verses that were guaranteed to make cancer cells spontaneously combust when uttered with absolute faith and sincerity. I probably nodded and smiled, for, although I don't believe faith works exactly like that, I knew she was concerned for my well-being and truly wanted to help.

Cancer patients have odd, uncomfortable conversations like this all the time. People seem to save their most haphazard comments for those battling cancer. And, quite often, the outcome is simultaneously hilarious and horrifying, for everyone involved.

People mean well. (Grandma surely did.) They want to show they care. They want to say meaningful words. They want to give you their wise observations on life, to fix things if you will, and then get the hell out of there.

But cancer is the proverbial square peg that doesn't fit into a ten minute conversational hole. It's too big, too surreal—a hopelessly difficult subject with way too many unanswerable questions attached. People often underestimate that fact when they offer comfort to someone who's hurting.

Let's be honest. We've all screwed up our share of conversations, despite our best intentions. I know I have. That's just part of life.

I Survived Cancer...

But perhaps conversations like this should be approached carefully, respectfully, like one approaches a minefield. Whether it's cancer, divorce, addictions, or whatever, the "answers" to whatever your friend or loved one is facing will likely come, eventually, little by little, as life moves along.

It's a process, not a pep-talk.

As my friend Don says, "First, do no harm." That's great advice. It's better to just show up at the door with an encouraging smile and a listening ear.

Oh yes. And write this down: *It never hurts to bring coconut crème pie.*

LANCE, A LOT

He smirks from the book jacket
having whipped cancer's sorry butt
and those skinny European bikers
in the French countryside
            seven times over.

His book's sold a gazillion copies
so he smirks and publishes, grants
interviews, gets clean bills of health.
He rides and wins and dates celebrities
            and smirks again.

His new book? Doing well, natch.
And why the heck not? He's driven!
Plus he leads a charmed life,
as big as his home country,
            TEXAS.

I won a city-wide 100 yard dash—
in fifth grade. I'm also trying to
beat cancer, again. I've written a book too!
My friends have promised to read it
            if it's published.

The hills are alive with success
and victory, triumph and prosperity,
with a rosy future and smirks.
But for those in the peleton,
            a mountain's waiting.

3

Ménage à Trois

Great looking nurses are a myth. Like mermaids, they're an interesting thought, but in all reality a hoax.

Oh sure, we've seen them on television shows and movies. Tune in to E.R., late night Cinemax, or practically any soap opera, and you see them all the time. But walk the halls of a hospital and...*nada*.

I'm speaking from experience. During my many hospital stays, I have been, without exception, assigned either: (1) the skinny, extremely nice, but rather mousy nurse; (2) the large, jovial Julia Child sort; or (3) the loud militant Patton variety, which can come in any shape or size. They are all competent and helpful, angels in disguise. But when it's time for a sponge bath, count me out.

Oh, I want to believe the attractive ones are out there. I really do. But it's like believing in Santa Claus: the older you get, the more doubtful you become.

Of course, I know I'm wrong about this. Just like there are black holes somewhere out in space, there are surely attractive nurses, too. I mean, think of the odds. Great looking nurses simply cannot be a figment of our collective imaginations.

But if they do exist, they must work in children's wards or urology departments or with podiatrists or something. Someplace I've never been. And unless it's the anesthesia talking, I'm pretty sure they avoid orthopedic hospitals and cancer centers altogether.

But who really cares if nurses are less than stunning?

Not me. I'm a happily married man, you see, with a wonderfully attractive wife! It's not like I'm so superficial as to be disappointed by an endless parade of Plain Janes in my hospital room. It's the statistical improbabilities that I find so fascinating. Really!

But still, one Pamela Anderson in an all-white outfit would lift the spirits a bit. They say that keeping a positive attitude counts for a lot when you're sick.

Strangely enough, this same phenomenon doesn't apply to female doctors, doctor's assistants, and therapist types. How do I know?

Well, stick with me.

In September of 2001, I had a small tumor removed from the triceps muscle of my right arm. It was cancerous, aggressive, and showed signs of spreading. So I was recommended for radiation therapy at a nearby hospital. I would leave my office an hour early, drive to the hospital, and have my arm zapped just like that.

Now if you're anything like me (and chances are you're not), radiation treatments are one of those things you have often heard discussed, but know absolutely nothing about.

What in the world is "radiation?" Is it a pill you take? A cream you rub in? A vat of glowing green liquid into which you are lowered? Is it some mysterious chamber you enter, wearing an aluminum suit? Is a nuclear reactor involved?

What exactly is going on here?

Well, I'm no doctor, but in my experience radiation therapy is very much like getting an x-ray. You know the routine. The dentist points a small gun-looking device at your jaw and takes a snapshot of the roots of your molars. The doctor puts your leg under a machine, and two seconds later someone can see the fracture.

For cancer patients undergoing radiation therapy, the apparatus is much bigger than your standard x-ray machine, but it essentially does the same thing. However, instead of a quick fraction of a second snapshot, the machine stays on for about twenty continuous seconds.

For the sarcoma in my upper arm, I was zapped from elbow to under-arm. First from the top of the arm and then from underneath.

It's really not so bad. You're locked inside an isolated lead-lined room, and a few minutes later, after the machine has completed its work, you're free to go. (Radiation patients usually do this for six weeks, only skipping weekends.)

The primary, short-term side effects are fatigue and burned skin. I was always very sleepy following my treatments, but after a brief power nap, I would feel pretty darn good. That is, until the fifth week. At that point, my skin really started to burn, like the worst sunburn of my life.

This is fairly common. After all, radiation is designed to kill any re-maining bad cells in you by essentially cooking them. Fortunately, the burns tend to heal nicely after a couple of painful weeks.

Of course, radiation treatments are not something to be taken too lightly. Radiation changes the molecular structure of the cells in your body per-manently. I was told that if my arm ever breaks, it would probably never heal. And, as you're probably aware, in large doses, radiation can cause cancer all by itself. So you don't want to radiate any area that doesn't ab-solutely need to be radiated.

In my case, the doctors wanted to radiate my upper arm, but for obvi-ous reasons not my internal organs or my head (although some have said that would have been a positive thing). This meant placing my arm as far from my chest as possible, but not too close to my head—somewhere comfortably in between. Plus, my arm had to be in the same position each time.

To accomplish this, I had to have a plastic body mold made of my back, shoulders, and right arm. During treatments, I would lie shirtless in the mold atop an operating table, with the radiation machine towering over me. The mold kept my arm in the exact same place each day.

The doctor in charge of radiation therapy was a woman from Switzerland or Sweden or some nearby European country with high mountains. She was about forty-five and fairly attractive, in a mysterious European sort of way. (She had the Swedish accent and everything.) I can't remember her first name, but I'll call her Frida, like the singer from Abba.

Now Frida was nice-looking, but her thirty-year old assistant, a blonde who may have been named Wendy, was a real knockout, the sort of person you find yourself trying to impress, simply to see if you can. (I seem to remember mentioning to her that I write film reviews for several newspapers. In response, Wendy just smiled her extremely white smile back at me, as if to say, "That's great. Now, can we get this over with, cancer guy?")

Wendy was in charge of making my body mold.

Now I've never been completely at ease when asked to go commando or shirtless before any medical personnel, male or female. I mean, it's just not natural, walking around without a shirt on or in one of those open hospital gowns, having normal conversations like some sort of male stripper. I was never one of those "take my shirt off" kind of guys. If God had intended us to walk around topless all the time, he wouldn't have made nipples.

Taking my shirt off so Frida, my doctor, could examine my arm was somewhat bothersome, but to be expected. However, taking it off for Wendy—the attractive blond assistant—that was way outside my comfort zone. If I had known that was coming, I might have done some crunches and side bends. But hindsight is twenty/twenty...

As for the body mold itself, it had a bean bag quality. Wendy explained that I would lie down on top of the mold, which would then conform to the shape of my body. After that, she had some way of fixing the mold in that position forever.

At this point, Wendy asked me to remove my shirt. I reluctantly obliged, thinking all the while about how I'd meant to start lifting weights. To make matters worse, as soon as I was topless, a female oncologist—not Wendy or Frida—stepped in the door. (Let's call her Leslie, for I once knew a Leslie who was pretty attractive.)

Leslie was in charge of determining the precise amount of radiation I would receive. She held a chart filled with what looked like calculus figures, and she recorded important information from me, as I shifted about uncomfortably in my shirtless state.

I tried to concentrate on Leslie's questions, but it was cold in there, and I was half naked. Plus, I kept wondering why all the workers in this place were females. That was so unfair!

Did I mention that Leslie was also attractive? She was. Not a real looker like Wendy, but she was the sexiest one of the three. Leslie was smart and funny, slim and brown-haired. Plus, for some inexplicable reason, she had left several buttons open on her shirt, showing more than just a hint of cleavage. Not that I really looked, mind you. As Jerry once told George on *Seinfeld*, "Looking at cleavage is like looking at the sun. You don't stare at it, it's too risky. You just get a sense of it, and then you look away."

I was definitely getting a sense of it.

Leslie mentioned she would be assisting Wendy with the body mold because "arms are tricky." I said, "Oh," in a state that was somewhere between panic and nirvana. I was having trouble adjusting to the fact that I would be lying on an operating table, topless, while two attractive females helped fit me into a body mold. The whole thing sounded grotesque and yet strangely exciting. I think I saw something like it once in a movie... when I was in college.

Things didn't go well. Apparently Wendy and Leslie needed the mold to fit very tightly around my arm and back area, but gravity had its own ideas and was diligently working against a tight fit. This left Wendy and Leslie with the task of adjusting the darn thing by pushing it up against me. They had to use their shoulders and bodies to achieve this affect.

But the poor gals just couldn't get a satisfactory fit by themselves. Wendy had to call for reinforcements: Frida and Karen, another cute assistant who suffered from a malady I will refer to here as "extreme top-heaviness." Poor girl.

I guess Wendy felt we needed two more babes in order to make the circus complete.

There I was, lying on the table, while three attractive women pushed and pushed against the mold so it would fit tightly around my naked form. (Frida stood by watching, as if to make sure nothing funny happened.) All three of them were literally pressed against me in a way that seemed borderline obscene.

I loved it! All sorts of naughty ideas passed through my mind.

"We've about got it," Leslie said. "Just a little bit more."

And then Leslie got a bright idea. In order to make the mold just a bit tighter, she reached across me and pulled on the other side of the mold. In other words, Leslie was now lying on top and across me, apologizing all the while, squeezing me into the mold. Wendy and Karen followed suit, and I was suddenly in a medical sandwich, the bacon in a BLT. I had two, and sometimes three, girls pressing, leaning over, or actually lying across or upon my naked torso, as Frida did whatever it took to fix the mold in place.

It was then that I realized I was experiencing one of the truly strange moments of my life, one I would likely never see again. It was like some sort of orgiastic dream, and I should have relaxed and tried to enjoy it while it lasted.

But in reality, it was all rather awkward and embarrassing, not just for me, but for the women as well, especially Wendy, Karen, and Leslie, who appeared to be making a move on me right there. Meanwhile, I was doing my best to avoid looking at Leslie's cleavage, which, after careful consideration, was less than six inches from my eyes!

I wanted to commemorate this bizarre moment with a few words. A toast. Something funny and a little outrageous to capture the moment forever. Something to make us all laugh about how strange life is. Something to take the edge off.

At first, I thought about saying, "I had a dream like this the other night..."

But then I came up with something better. I would say, "Hey now! Nobody said anything about *ménage à trois* treatments!"

Yes, it was a pretty funny line. But it was also highly inappropriate, the kind of statement that could conceivably offend someone or cause a lawsuit to be filed. Risky, yes, but the payoff could be huge if they thought it was funny, too.

What if one of them didn't have a sense of humor?

Hmmm.... What should I do?

Under normal circumstances, I would never pass up the chance to make a good joke, regardless of the consequences. But these weren't normal circumstances. These attractive women were going to be pointing a huge radiation shooting machine at me over the next two months. What if one of them had an abusive boyfriend or had a bad ménage à trois experience in her past, and this was the one comment that sent her over the edge?

I kept my mouth shut that day. But I still think it was one of the best lines I never said.

PARTING WORDS

So it's come down to this.
Well, you know what they say,
death and taxes...
     (this is met with silence)

Uh-hum. I suppose this will be
my last chance to say
something important,
to let you all know how I truly feel...
     (sweat forms on his brow)

I've tried to speak my mind
over the years, within reason. And so,
if I have something that really needs
to be said—to clear the air if you will
or to pass down some words of wisdom—
now would definitely be the time...
     (he looks around in vain for water)

Funny though, phrases like "go forth
and prosper" and "all you need is love"
aren't doing it for me just now.
     (he taps his fingers nervously)

For some reason, all I can think of
is how Salma Hayek was nominated
for Best Actress.
     (he exits, stage left)

     I Survived Cancer...

4

Anesthesiologists

Anesthesiologists.

Who would have thought they would be such characters, the class clowns, court jesters, and sadistic bullies of the hospital? Not me. I would have put money on plastic surgeons or perhaps urologists.

But then again, anesthesiologists do have the power of the IV. They can put you to sleep for as long as they darn well please, and who knows what is going on in the meantime? The situation is fraught with uncomfortable possibilities, especially if you've randomly drawn a practical joker.

I saw on the news one day that a doctor was being sued because he carved his initials onto a patient's uterus during an operation, thus giving a new meaning to the term "inside joke."

Perhaps that's the kind of tricks anesthesiologists play once patients are sedated. Perhaps they dress us up like Elvis or Marilyn Monroe. Maybe they curl our hair, put rouge on our cheeks, and paint our toenails, just for a few laughs. Perhaps they make comments about our bodies, about shrinkage and cellulite and such. Maybe they take revealing photographs of us while we are unconscious and then post them on some bizarre anesthesiologist website.

Who really knows?

If my anesthesiologist takes a sudden disliking to me, what's to prevent him or her from "upping" the dose, so I become violently ill upon regaining consciousness? Or, even worse, I might receive too little medicine—

enough to be semi-conscious, still capable of feeling pain.

My first experience with an anesthesiologist should have alerted me to the fact that they are...quirky. I was scheduled for shoulder surgery as a result of a high school football injury and would be on the operating table for several hours. This was before arthroscopic surgery became so common, and I was about to be the proud recipient of a six-inch scar.

To be honest, I don't remember much about my anesthesiologist, but I do know he knocked me out for an incredibly long time. I've always been a lightweight when it comes to medicine. What causes one person to become slightly drowsy causes me to go into a deep slumber. But in this case, the result was hibernation.

Many hours after my surgery was over, I was awakened by a loud authoritative nurse (see Chapter 3) saying it was time for me to get up and go to the bathroom. I had been asleep for "much too long."

I tried to protest, saying I was nauseous and couldn't possibly make it to the bathroom. But she went into Patton-mode and yanked me into a sitting position.

I responded to this breach of protocol by launching a projectile stream of vomit all over both of us. And I do mean all over—imagine Linda Blair after a Thanksgiving feast.

For some reason, the nurse was less than thrilled by my little offering, and so she sought her revenge during the clean-up phase. With a smirk, she reached and yanked off my hospital nightgown, leaving me naked on the bed and without sufficient control over my anesthesia-ridden body to do anything about it. She then left to clean herself off and grab a camera.

I was alone and helpless and completely commando. I remember trying to find something to cover myself, but I was having trouble staying awake, thanks to my anesthetic hangover.

About that time, I heard my parents outside the door, talking to...someone. Now who was that? I could almost recognize the voice, but not quite.

Then it came to me—they were speaking to our pastor. And the trio was about to enter my room!

What happened from there? All I know for sure is that I passed out just as things were getting interesting. When I awoke sometime later, I was in a fresh hospital gown.

I've never had the nerve to ask my parents if they entered my room with our pastor to find me lying there naked and garnished with vomit. But I'd really like to think they somehow avoided that unpleasant scene, for everyone's sake.

And where was the anesthesiologist who had brought me to this nearly comatose state? Who knows? After the assault, he made a complete getaway.

My next anesthesiologist experience came during childbirth, when my wife was giving birth to our daughter Madison. The anesthesiologist, Dr. G, had a sparkling reputation, for the medical team kept telling LeAnn how lucky she was to have him.

Dr. G was the happiest, smilingest guy I had ever seen. His never-ending grin convinced me that he loved his job more than anyone in the world. Either that or he'd been in some industrial accident that had permanently fixed his face that way. I'd opt for the first choice, if forced to, but one never really knows.

When the time was ripe, Dr. G smiled, administered an epidural to LeAnn, and then left. After that I didn't see him for quite a while. I suppose he was off doing his smiling magic for others too, for we were not the only expectant parents that day.

He emerged later, however, just as Madison's head was crowning. I was, of course, fairly busy at the time, and so I only noted his sudden appearance at this glorious—but seemingly private—moment in our lives. But as Madison fully emerged and we discovered she was a she, I saw Dr. G standing there beaming at me, as if he himself had participated in the fathering of this child.

And he wasn't alone.

I guess Dr. G had the right to be there, staring at my wife's holy of holies;

he was a participant on the medical team, after all. But who were these people with him? I think there were three, possibly four, people I had never seen before in my life. Like Dr. G, they appeared to be of Middle Eastern descent, and they were all standing and smiling in the direction of my wife's "region."

Were these fellow anesthesiologists? Trainees? Family members? Or just some curious passersby? It was hard to say, but I got the feeling Dr. G knew them and had, in fact, invited them to the party.

As Madison was handed to me, Dr. G waved good-bye and gave me a thumbs-up sign. I think I did the same back, for he was our anesthesiologist and would soon be sending a bill my way. He and his mysterious entourage disappeared, never to be seen again.

My next memorable anesthesiologist encounter came after knee surgery. I was scheduled to have some screws removed from an earlier operation. During pre-surgical consultations, my anesthesiologist recommended a spinal block, a procedure that is similar to an epidural. He said this was my best option, and the most common side effect was a headache.

I agreed to the procedure, because, well, I don't have a medical degree. And so, off we went. The anesthesiologist placed a needle in my spine, and in a minute or so I had no feeling at all below my waist. I was able to lie there and watch, fully conscious, as they cut open my knee and removed the screws. What a strange ride!

About two hours later, when the surgery was over and the feeling in my legs had returned, I was given the okay to leave the hospital. I decided to head to the bathroom before the 45-minute trip home. "Be prepared," as they say in the scouts, although I was never actually in the scouts.

I entered the bathroom, headed to the urinal, and unzipped my fly. I then reached down to commence urination proceedings, but my you-know-what WASN'T THERE! "Oh my God," I wailed. "That idiot cut off my penis!"

I ran to the mirror, scared to death of what I would not see. But to my great relief, I had not been turned into a Eunuch.

I Survived Cancer...

But still, something was very wrong. I had no sensation down there. I mean, the feeling in my legs had returned a half hour earlier. Why was this place any different?

Oh my God, I thought. *They severed the nerve to my penis!* I would remain in this dead wood state for all of eternity. My sex life was now a thing of the past. That consent form I signed never mentioned this possibility.

But perhaps this was just a temporary setback. Maybe in an hour or so, everything would be back in order down there.

I wanted to ask my anesthesiologist about it, but just couldn't. The subject was too embarrassing, and I was in a state of near panic. Plus, I would find out shortly whether or not I was okay. If I asked my anesthesiologist, he would probably have me drop my drawers so he could make sure everything was progressing well. I could avoid this, possibly, by keeping my mouth shut.

By the time I got home, I was pleased to find that everything had returned to normal. I let out a nervous breath and relaxed. "Everything is going to be fine," I thought, as I began developing the worst migraine headache of my life. It was as if a heavy metal band was living inside my brain and was trying, as best as they could, to make my head explode by cranking up the noise louder and LOUDER!

But at least I had my penis.

During my first ordeal with cancer, the anesthesiologist saga continued. I was awaiting surgery in Houston when one of the nurses informed me that my anesthesiologist would be "Dr. R." She then rolled her eyes, as if to say, sarcastically, "lucky you."

Dr. R turned out to be the loudest and most abrasive human being I have ever met. You could hear him approaching long before he reached my bed, like Darth Vader or thunder before a summer storm. One got the sense that Dr. R liked people to know he was there.

He introduced himself, in his coarse lumberjack way, and I answered his questions as best I could for someone in my condition. Most importantly, I recounted my unpleasant anesthesia history.

As he pretended to listen, Dr. R began preparing my IV. He then began firing off questions about my current profession.

"So...you're a lawyer, is that right?" he asked, as he pulled a large needle from his secret drawer.

"Uh, yeah," I responded. Oh great. We were going to do the lawyer conversation. I would be stuck in more ways than one.

"What type of law do you practice?" he said, asking the next standardized question from the conversationally challenged doctor's handbook.

"Well, I'm a lawyer for one of the Judges on the Oklahoma Court of Criminal Appeals. I write opinions for the Court, do research, stuff like that," I answered.

"Oh, so you're a law clerk," he offered.

Now we don't use the words "law clerk" where I work. That has derogatory connotations. Law clerks are normally understood to be lawyers fresh out of law school, young pups who work for a judge for a few years and then move on to real jobs. To call me a law clerk was like calling a meteorologist a weatherman.

I tried to explain this to Dr. R. "No, not really a law clerk. I'm a Judicial Assistant. I mean, these are good jobs, not ones people drop after a year or two. You can't even get hired there unless you have five years experience in the legal system."

"But it's still just a clerkship, right?" he fired back with a grin on his face.

"Well, it's not some temporary training program or anything like that. It's a legitimate job. Hardly anyone ever leaves."

"How old are you?" he asked.

"Thirty-seven."

"Wow. And you're still a law clerk..."

At this point, the unpleasant conversation ended, because I had cried out in pain as he thrust the IV needle deep into my vain in his contentious way.

I Survived Cancer...

And so, Dr. R was sort of a bully. I had the distinct impression he was always measuring me up so he could knock me down a bit later. Not normal bedside manner for a doctor, I suppose, but he seemed to like it.

The last time I saw him was on the day after my surgery, following approximately twelve straight hours of vomiting. Dr. R was upbeat and wholly unapologetic about my condition, as he again challenged my manhood. "You're really a lightweight," he said. "I gave you less anesthesia than any other patient I've ever had, and you still wouldn't wake up after surgery. It was like a pediatric dose, swear to God."

I can't remember how I responded. Nor can I tell you the things I was thinking about him right then, or the things I said about him just after he had left, or the things I thought about him just now.

One of my most recent anesthesiologists was either the most accomplished and adventurous man I have ever met, or he was a bold-faced liar.

His name was Dr. H, and he seemed friendly enough. He was short and stocky, which tends to corroborate what he told my wife and I, that he was a college wrestler many years ago. *Wow, my anesthesiologist is a former wrestler,* I thought. I was truly impressed.

"After that, I was a practicing veterinarian for ten years," he offered with a straight face.

"You were?" I asked. This, too, was impressive. Not only was he a doctor, he was also a college wrestler and a vet!

I must admit, however, that the whole vet thing gave me pause. I began wondering whether or not he would do something really unconventional, like placing my IV into my calf or neck. Perhaps he would recommend some medicine that was "experimental," but only in people.

He did, in fact, place my IV in a much lower part of my arm than I was accustomed to, but his handiwork seemed to work quite well. So I relaxed a bit.

"Yeah, then I got tired of that, so I moved to Alaska and did the Iditarod." He said this as if it was no strange thing. Meanwhile, I began looking around for the hidden cameras and Alan Funt.

"You did the...Iditarod? Are you kidding?" I asked.

"No, of course not. Well, at first I was just there on the medical team to look after the dogs, but then I actually completed the race on my third year."

I really didn't know how to respond to this. Doctor, wrestler, veterinarian, and Iditarod racer. What was next? Was he an astronaut, too? Perhaps he had helped create the Internet. I was afraid to ask any more questions, for fear he might tell me he once played Curly in the Broadway production of *Oklahoma!*

Dr. H seemed to be ultra-curious about life, one of those guys who could only stand to be in a job for five years or so before moving on to the next great achievement. He was thoroughly fascinated when I told him I was a movie critic and had seen hundreds of movies over the last several years.

"Wow! A film critic. That's got to be one of the greatest jobs in the world!" he said. "You know, I have a collection of 10,000 DVDs at home."

Oh, brother. Now he had a massive DVD library, too. I made a note to myself to call the newspapers I write for, just to make sure he hadn't submitted his resume. On paper, I could never compete with him for a job.

Dr. H was also quite the jokester. I can't give you many examples, because most of them occurred as the anesthesia began surging through my body. But I do recall one thing he said just after I was wheeled into the operating room.

I was quite drowsy by that time, but I remember how cold the room was, something like fifty degrees. A kind, but not pretty, nurse offered me an extra blanket, and I willingly took her up on the offer.

As she began tucking the blanket under me, Dr. H looked me in the eyes and said, "Ahhh...a nice warm blanket. We want to make sure you're all covered up. If there's one thing about this place, we respect your privacy..."

That was comforting, I thought.

But then he added, "until you're asleep."

I winced as his words confirmed my suspicions. Who knew what games they were getting ready to play with me? Perhaps my surgery would soon be added to his DVD collection. I would be video #10,001.

INSOMNIAC

The doctor cuts a mean scar.
People often spot the carvings
in my flesh and comment
on the craftsmanship.
"Ooh, nice job," they say.

The doctor is articulate, reads
Marquez, attended the right schools
and works at a great hospital.
The doctor's up-to-speed
on my condition.

But the doctor doesn't know
where Oklahoma is.
And the doctor's favorite film
is *Dude, Where's My Car?*
And sleep thus eludes me.

5

I've Got Mail

I received a letter in the mail the other day. That's right, a letter. It had one of those little stamps on it and everything.

Normally, I don't receive letters. People just don't write them like they used to. Now they send emails, which are kind of like letters, except they're trimmed down to one or two cryptic sentences, nouns and punctuation optional. I receive plenty of those.

Even when people did write letters, not so many years ago, I was rarely a recipient. I guess I wasn't too good at returning the favor. Oddly enough, letter writers tend to frown on that sort of thing. They write and expect you to write back. I rarely did. And so, my mailbox was usually empty, except for bills and junk mail.

After I was diagnosed with cancer, letters came in fairly regularly. I suppose it's because letters provide a safe distance for people who want to show their concern, but at the same time avoid getting too close to all that icky grief and depression.

I mean, cancer is so...awkward. Very few people know exactly what to do with the news that a friend or loved one has the disease. There's such a fine line between showing concern and pissing someone off. So we tend to err on the side of giving those hurting their "space."

With a letter, however, you can make contact, say a few kind words, give some advice if you feel so inclined, and then get the hell out, job well done. (Let's see, I can cross "comforting Aunt Margaret" off my To Do list.)

Even now, many months after my last surgery, when I am hopefully cured for the umpteenth time, letters keep trickling in. And it's often quite surprising when I find out who wrote them. Some people you think will surely send you a letter never do. Cancer freaked them out so badly that they took a vow of silence. But others, people you haven't thought about in decades, send a letter out of the blue, often saying the kindest, heartfelt words.

Unless they have some sort of agenda.

One of my more memorable letters came from a person I barely know, one of the charismatic, faith-healing persuasion. Even though our relationship has, to date, consisted of tossing a few footballs more than a decade ago and approximately forty-five minutes of light conversation, this virtual stranger suddenly resurfaced a few months back with hopes of shedding some much-needed heavenly light my way.

Now don't get me wrong. I believe in God and feel certain that many people have experienced what can only be described as a miracle, insofar as their health is concerned. I pray to God often about many things, including my battle with cancer. And I believe God is able to heal me, if so desired. After all, God is...God. Healing is part of the job description.

It's just that I think God tends to use skilled doctors, educated health-care professionals, and advanced state-of-the-art equipment to accomplish healing in most circumstances. And sometimes, despite one's strong faith in God, that desired healing never comes.

Oh, I want to be healed as much as the next guy. You can trust me on that. I'm like Linus waiting for the Great Pumpkin in the pumpkin patch: I'm trying to be as sincere about becoming cancer-free as possible.

But still, I don't think there are any guarantees.

I've never quite bought in to the theology that says a perfect healing awaits every person who utters the proper prayer in the right frame of mind. There's something suspiciously non-miraculous about a sure thing, the Jabez prayer that obligates God to perform a miracle when all the correct words are said with utmost sincerity. If that's the way the world works, then we're in control of our own destinies, and God has just been miracled right out of business.

Besides, why should God miraculously heal me (or anyone else) of cancer when there are hundreds of qualified physicians out there—including the most skilled oncologists in the world—just waiting to do the same? Why deprive so many young well-educated men and women of a much-deserved paycheck?

But I'm getting ahead of myself.

"Dear Jimmy Lee," the letter began. Some people who have known me since childhood still call me Jimmy Lee, even though I switched to Jim decades ago and have never used my middle name. It's an Oklahoma-style term of endearment, I guess, although it actually has the opposite effect.

The letter continued. "I was reading this article by _____ the other day, and I believe God spoke to my heart to make a copy for you. I pray God's perfect will for your life, which is complete healing. God bless." The person then signed the letter, which is itself a miracle, given the article's subject matter and tone.

The article was supposedly written by a television evangelist, one of those guys in expensive suits you can watch on Sunday morning, if you are into that sort of thing. (I'm not.) As for this particular televangelist—or for that matter any other—I didn't know much about him. Beyond the bad haircut and all-knowing attitude, his life and background were, for me, a blank page.

Upon closer inspection, however, it appeared that the article was not actually written by the televangelist, but by his wife. I found this intriguing, for Almighty God had reportedly instructed my letter-writing friend to send me the article, but had, at the same time, allowed my friend to be mistaken about who had written the darn thing. Such errancy seems so, well, un-Godlike.

But again, I digress.

I won't summarize the entire article for you. But it began by asking the following: Have you been unable to receive your healing due to a lack of faith?

This was the article that God had told my letter-writing friend to send my way? Ouch!

Apparently, that's me. The sad cancer patient who hasn't received the healing that's out there waiting on me because of my shameful lack of faith.

You might wonder how the person who sent me this article—this letter-writer whom I've only seen once or twice in the last ten years and who lives many miles away—was able to know I was suffering from lack of faith. Well, my cancer had recently returned, hadn't it? That's proof in the pudding. These things don't happen to Mother Theresa or Billy Graham.

Or do they?

The faith-healing logic goes something like this: Everyone in the history of mankind who has ever died of any prolonged sickness—be it cancer, heart disease, Alzheimer's, AIDS, the plague, typhoid, or the common flu—has suffered from this same incurable spiritual malady as me, i.e., pathetically weak faith. True God believers never die from sickness, although they do die in their sleep from natural causes (Abraham, Moses), in sudden devil-devised catastrophes (Job's family), in unfortunate wars (Jonathon), in birthing a child (Rachel), as crime victims (Abel, Stephen), or as wrongly accused prisoners (Jesus and most of his disciples). Apparently, God's desired prosperity for my life doesn't cover these sorts of random calamities.

So what about those God-believers who suffer the indignities of paralysis, blindness, mental illness, rheumatoid arthritis, chronic pain, heart failure, or cancer? What happens to them? Well, according to my friend, if they are able to muster enough faith, they receive their "complete healing" (Bartimaeus) or they are raised from the dead (Lazarus).

Those who can't exercise enough faith are, like me, in big trouble.

Of course, I'm alive and kicking, up to this point anyway. There's still hope for me yet. I guess that explains why I've received so many self-help books dealing with faith healing and miracles since my cancer diagnosis.

Like Job, I seem to be a poster-child for guilt-inducing advice, a bulls-eye for those with spiritual darts to throw.

For example, somebody once sent me the book, *Christ the Healer,* a self-proclaimed classic by the late F.F. Bosworth. Although I never read it, I did skim through its pages, thus allowing some of its bullying promises to punch me hard in the gut.

One of the more memorable chapters describes the various reasons why people don't experience healing. Some of those include: ignorance of the Bible; overeating; an evil spirit within; unconfessed sin; an unwillingness to surrender to God; and, you've got it, lack of faith.

I wonder which one of these was the downfall of my great-grandfather, a great Christian man who died a horrible death from brain cancer many years ago. He sometimes cheated at cards, if I remember right, by talking across the table to my great-grandmother. Perhaps God didn't approve.

Or how about a pastor in my community who faithfully served his church for more than forty years and was reportedly loved and respected by the entire city? As he was dying a horrible cancer death, I'm told he came to the conclusion that he'd been given the "ministry of pain." Was this an evil spirit talking? Perhaps he'd eaten too many helpings of mashed potatoes at the homes of church members who had invited him for Sunday dinner.

Plus, I wonder how F.F. Bosworth and all the other faith healers died. If it had anything to do with a virus, a weakened immune system, congestive heart failure, or the gout, then I'm confused.

But let's move on, for my point is certainly not to disprove miraculous healings or to poke fun at those who've figured out the magic formula. My point is to simply suggest that healing is not an absolute given. And if that is true, then it follows that anyone who tells you that healing is absolutely guaranteed when you've exercised enough faith is committing a form of spiritual abuse, well-intended or not.

I shudder to think of all the people over the years who have had their spirits absolutely crushed by the faith-healing bullies of the world. How many have died with the words "My God, my God, why have you forsaken me" on their lips?

When I was in the hospital last year, I was given a copy of a little book that dealt with faith-healing and cancer. The book tells of the author's seemingly miraculous healing from incurable liver cancer that threatened to take her life a few short weeks after diagnosis. Rather than seek medical intervention that might slightly prolong her days—for there was no cure—the author reportedly headed home. She and her husband (a televangelist) prayed and the cancer disappeared. She shares some of the verses she prayed and her conclusion that she had been healed by the word of God. The book ends with letters from physicians confirming the miracle.

While that is a great story, one I sincerely hope is true, I doubt it is a typical result for most diagnosed with liver cancer, even for those who diligently pray for healing from God, using all the correct techniques and suggested verses. Of course, I have no data to back this up, other than the common knowledge that everyone who is ever born into this world eventually dies, and most of those from some sort of physical infirmity. (This includes the author's televangelist husband, who reportedly died from a heart attack a few years ago.)

Did you know that more than 700,000 Americans die each year from heart disease? Another 550,000 die each year from cancer. Approximately 300,000 die from strokes, aneurisms, and respiratory illnesses. 70,000 or so die from diabetes, and 65,000 are victims of the flu. Another 50,000 die from Alzheimer's.

Indeed, of the top eight causes of death in the United States, all but one of them (accidents) are the result of illness.

Is it really possible that every one of these victims (more than 1.7 million) died because they did not have enough faith to receive their healing? What are the odds that there wasn't a man or woman of faith among the lot?

And how about the more than 1,000 children under the age of four who die in this country each year from the same causes? Did they not say their goodnight prayers? Did they eat too much formula?

Based upon the people I have known who died from sickness or disease, along with the statistical realities listed above, I find it quite easy to conclude that God allows some people of faith to never be physically healed, this side of heaven.

The problem, however, is that this flawed healing theology has enough truth behind it to make someone who has cancer feel very uncomfortable and confused. The Bible has dozens of stories of healing. Healing was unquestionably one of Jesus' main things. I'm not sure you can find a single example of a time when he refused to heal someone who was sick or suffering from a serious physical condition.

What would Jesus do? Why, he would heal them, of course. That is, unless they didn't have enough faith. In light of what may be read about the life and compassionate heart of Jesus, I can see how a person might conclude that God intends every person in the world to be totally free from sickness and disease.

That's the rub, you see, the painful, spiritually based, and well-intended suggestion that hits nearly every cancer patient smack in the face. In matters of theology, cancer seems to be hopelessly connected to a person's faith or lack thereof.

But perhaps we should look just a little bit further.

As much as we want to fight against the notion, my glance through the newspaper each day convinces me that this isn't heaven, that hoped-for place where sickness and death are no more.

In fact, the Bible has plenty of stories about people of faith suffering. Job was a righteous man who was given boils from head to foot. When his friends insinuated the innocent do not suffer, God chastised them for not speaking "what is right." Rachel died giving birth to Benjamin. The prophet Elisha died of a protracted illness. Lazarus, one of Jesus' close friends, died from a sickness. His faith did not save him. Paul, one of the most devout men to ever walk on this earth, complained of a "thorn in the flesh." He prayed three times for God to heal him of this infirmity, but no healing came. Paul's conclusion: God desired this condition so that Paul would not exalt himself. Even Jesus described himself as one who was familiar with suffering.

There are plenty of other examples from well-known spiritual leaders. Billy Graham suffers from Parkinson's disease. Augustine died of a wasting disease. Martin Luther died a difficult death following a series of illnesses.

And let's not forget Mother Theresa. She died from a heart attack, God rest her soul, following a long battle with heart disease. This was a condition that affected her for years, as her own good deeds will affect the world for years to come.

Matthew 5:45 says that God "causes His sun to rise on the evil and the good, and sends rain on the righteous and unrighteous." In other words, bad things happen to good people, and good things happen to bad people. There are no guarantees of a life free of illness. We are all on an even playing field.

Unfortunately, the topic of faith-healing and cancer is not strictly a matter of religion. Cancer sufferers are also challenged by nutritionists, who hit from a different angle. They tout miracle products that will save your cancerous life. They send books that speak of defeating cancer with nutrition, with, supposedly, an insider's viewpoint. These books don't beat you over the head with God. Instead, they preach a different gospel: you can outsmart your doctors with science, by eating the right foods, taking the right vitamins.

On the night before a particularly awful surgery, I was once called by a man I didn't know who begged me not to go through with a surgery that an entire board of oncologists had approved. He had a miracle pill that had "Nobel Science" behind it. It was by far the cruelest telephone call that I have ever received, perhaps even the cruelest event in my life.

I once asked my doctor what she thought about all this. She smiled and said, "Just take Centrum."

So I think I will. I will take these pills that are surely good for me, without placing all my hopes in a miracle to come my way. And I will continue praying with as much faith as I can. Studies show that having a positive attitude really can improve one's chances.

Perhaps God will heal me. Perhaps not. Perhaps God has other plans. But whatever the future holds, I'm going to do my best to face it with a spirit of willingness and trust, realizing all the while that I certainly haven't figured out everything.

I continue walking forward on this crazy path, wherever it leads. But I have to confess: I still struggle sometimes...

Especially when I open the mailbox.

UNABOMBERS

they send innocuous letters
sprinkled with encouraging words
and blessings that BLOW UP
in smiling faces, plunge deeply
into unsuspecting hearts

who knew these unabombers
filled their pens with deadly venom
oh how we've been fooled
thinking it was wholesome milk
dribbling down their chins

where do they recruit their disciples
and teach this prosperity terrorism
perhaps in some militia manifesto
home school elective
or suburban Sunday School

6

On the Road

Once the official word comes in, "yes, you have cancer," the world you once knew changes radically. Life becomes a frantic existence. Important and difficult decisions must be made constantly, one right after another, and the choices you make will significantly influence the rest of your tenuous life.

Now this is a problem if you're like me and sometimes struggle with making decisions, especially really big decisions. For with cancer, each decision seems to hinge on another while affecting several others at the same time. And there's no relief once a big decision is finally made. Cancer is like the Hydra: nearly every decision you dispose of generates two or three new ones.

I suppose it's a little bit like being lost in the middle of a jungle. Do you head north, south, east, or west? Just because you finally choose north doesn't mean you won't find a raging river, dangerous quicksand, or hungry tigers along your way.

For me, the official word came from a local orthopedic surgeon, a kind-hearted and not-so-young doctor who miraculously honed in on my problem and was ready to do some serious cutting on my arm, without delay. He had called me the day before with the bad news, and now my wife and I were sitting in his office, discussing the next step.

"Well, young man, what we need to do is remove the triceps muscle in that right arm there. That's the protocol anyway. It's a tough break for a thirty-seven year old, I know, but if we remove the triceps, you *should* be fine. I mean, you're going to have a bum arm and all, but you can live with that."

"What about chemotherapy and radiation?" I asked, for I was clueless about my prospects. Cancer always meant chemotherapy and radiation, didn't it?

"Well, we'll probably need to schedule you a visit with an oncologist at some point. I think he's on vacation this week, but never you mind. According to the literature, you don't treat this stuff with chemotherapy or radiation. This is basically a cutting deal." He said this in a matter-of-fact way.

A cutting deal. Those are tough words to process when they're coming from a surgeon, a man who is in the very business of cutting people open. A cutting deal was essentially his job description.

Sure he knew about opening someone up with a scalpel, but how much did he know about cancer? More specifically, *my* cancer? There was at least a decent chance he knew nothing at all.

And was there really only one oncologist in town, one who was...on vacation? I live in a fairly big city (100,000 people), but suddenly it seemed as though I were living in Mayberry.

My wife and I felt strongly that a second opinion was in order, a confirmation from some reliable specialist in the field, especially when we were discussing the reality of crippling my arm, making it much less effective at doing the sort of things arms do.

The only problem is you could probably count on one hand the doctors in Oklahoma who had ever seen a cancer of this type. I had an extremely rare form of cancer, a sarcoma called malignant fibrous hystiocytoma (MFH), which was even rarer because it was in my arm. Who was I supposed to call about my case? Dr. Phil?

Fortunately, we'd already started doing our homework. The night before my visit with the orthopedic surgeon, I had done some internet research and learned that M.D. Anderson in Houston, Texas (one of the

I Survived Cancer...

best cancer centers in the world with some of the best survival rates) had its own Sarcoma Center, one of the few such centers in the world. Houston is about a seven-hour drive from my home, not exactly a short trip, but do-able. LeAnn and I had already made the decision to head there, no matter the cost.

But now I had to break the news to the surgeon, this man who had been so helpful, so instrumental in my diagnosis. Here he was ready to cut on my arm next Wednesday, and I had to rain on his surgical parade. Poor guy.

I didn't know how to approach him. Would he be angry? Hurt? Rejected? Would he get defensive, or would he be understanding? This was beginning to feel a lot like a break-up, and I was never particularly good at those. I mean, I just couldn't let this local guy operate on my arm when I was seven hours away from one of the best cancer centers in the world. But I wasn't too wild about telling him.

I had to let him down easy.

So I commenced stall tactics.

"We're, uhhh, going to need some time to think this over...to discuss our options and everything. Maybe talk to someone who's seen this before. I mean, it's a big decision. We need to decide what's best for us."

"Oh...well, sure, take some time to talk it over," he said. "In the meantime, I'll make some arrangements..."

"Uh, okay," I squeaked, as I turned and gave my wife a weak smile.

LeAnn was looking at me incredulously, as if I were an alien that had just landed on earth. Stalling just wasn't in her vocabulary.

"What in the world are you talking about?" she asked aloud.

"Just, uhh, well, you know, um..." I replied. This is a common male response to such a direct attack, stringing together several nonsense words and then slinging them out there, hoping they will stick. Funny though, it has never been known to work.

"I'm sorry, doctor. I don't know why he said that. Listen, there's really nothing for us to talk over. We've already decided to go to M.D. Anderson.

So we need to pick up our records and documents." She glared at me with accusatory eyes.

I said, "Yeah, well, that and...yes. True."

The doctor was nice about the whole thing, although I think I detected a hint of disappointment. "Well, they'll certainly do you right down there. That's a top-notch outfit. Yessirree."

What a relief! He took it like a man. This wasn't his first breakup.

Moments later, some MRI photographs, biopsy results, radiology reports, and a few doctor's notes were handed to us, and we were sent on our merry way. We hadn't even called M.D. Anderson yet, but we were on our own. All ties with the locals had been severed.

Fortunately, I had no trouble getting M.D. Anderson to accept my case. After I sent them my MRI and biopsy report, I was in like Flynn. I had a rare case, you see, and that means the waiting list, for me, is not very long.

My appointment was in nine days. My doctor would be a young woman. This was a bit of a paradigm shift from the doctor we had just left. But my new doctor specialized in sarcoma. "She sees this all day long," I was told.

Another huge relief! Of course, the difficult decisions were far from over, for getting accepted by M.D. Anderson brought as many questions as it did answers.

Would my insurance plan cover my medical expenses there, or would they be treated "out-of-network," meaning I would be paying out the *whazoo*? What about the expenses going to Houston, i.e., hotel, meals, travel? Were those covered? Should we fly or drive? Flying is expensive, but you don't waste two days getting there and back. Of course, when you fly, you have to rent a car...

LeAnn and I flew to Houston the first couple of times, when I had my initial visit and then an extended stay for tests and surgery. Soon we learned that trips to Houston would become a regular part of our lives—at least one trip every three months for several years. So we decided driving would usually be our best option. A round trip takes about two and a half tanks of gas. And with the help of the internet, I've been able to get a few bargains at some nice hotels.

To a certain extent, my Houston road trips have been like living out a Hemingway novel or *On the Road with Jack Keroac,* with a little Roald Dahl or Tim Burton thrown in for good measure. LeAnn and I (and sometimes our kids) pack a few suitcases, load the car with drinks and snacks, and head to a sunnier place with as much cash as we can spare at the time.

We drive through such wondrous towns as Ardmore, Gainesville, Ennis, Corsicana, Fairfield, Centerville, Madisonville, and Huntsville. We stop and eat at whatever roadside restaurant looks good at the time. We cross over the Red River and pass by North Texas University, Dalley Plaza (where JFK was shot), the Huntsville prison, and a monstrous statue of Sam Houston. We read books, listen to tapes, and talk about life.

Once we actually arrive in Houston, these odd vacations become odder still, a strange mixture of fun and romance blended with the macabre. During the good days, we devote most of our time to sightseeing, movies, trips to the beach, shopping, eating at our favorite restaurants, and relaxing at the hotel pool. During the bad ones, I'm wearing a silly hospital gown and wristband as I wait in line for an MRI with a group of octogenarians.

Sometimes, my wife and kids are unable to go, so I head to Houston with one of my friends.

My friend John has traveled with me to Houston several times. During these trips, we've stayed with John's friends, the Rosses—who have graciously opened their home to me. I suppose Houston has many families who welcome M.D. Anderson patients into their homes. It is a wonderful ministry, and I am one of many who have been blessed by it.

Still, it's always a bit awkward, staying in another family's home, especially in the middle of the week. Your hosts must get up and go to work the next day, take their kids to school and soccer practice, and make dinner. No matter how hard they try to make you feel welcome, you tend to get in their way.

My first trip with John illustrates my point. We arrived before five, but the Rosses weren't due to be home until sometime after six. So we decided to catch a movie. I drove us to an art house theater I knew in the Montrose District. *The Closet* was playing there, and I really wanted to see it.

John, who's a bit homophobic, was less than thrilled about sitting beside his buddy in a Montrose art house theater, watching a subtitled French film about a man who pretends he is gay so he won't lose his job.

But what could he do? I had cancer.

After watching the film and grabbing a bite to eat, John and I drove to his friends' home. We arrived just after nine, and I was exhausted. I would have given anything to just walk in and hit the hay. But you can't do that when you're a guest. It would be rude.

John began catching up with the Rosses, while I sat politely on the couch, smiling as they reminisced about bygone days. I found myself drifting off several times, not because of the conversation, but because I was tired from all the cancer stress.

When midnight approached, John and his friends decided to call it a night. At this point, we were taken to our rooms. Due solely to proximity, John was awarded the visitor's room, while I lucked into the bedroom of my hosts' three-year old son.

Now I'm not being ungrateful, mind you, but John definitely got the better deal. (On the next trip, however, I evened the score.)

But I couldn't worry about who got the better room. My appointment was at 9:00 a.m. the next morning, and I needed some shut-eye. The Rosses live in far west Houston and rush-hour traffic anywhere in Houston is an absolute nightmare.

I slept fitfully that night. I had a lot on my mind, after all, and I was in a three year old's twin bed.

Unfortunately, I awoke too early, about 5:30 a.m. After ten minutes of trying to drift back to sleep, I gave up and headed for the bathroom.

Upon concluding my business, I opened the bathroom door and found the three-year old standing there. We hadn't met at this point, because he was already asleep when John and I arrived.

"Oh, I thought you were Uncle John," he said, clearly disappointed. This was an awkward moment, as I tried to think of a way to maneuver past the little guy so I could crawl back into his bed for twenty more minutes of sleep. But there was nowhere to go. He had me blocked.

And then, he noticed his bedroom light was on. He eyed me suspiciously. "Did you sleep in my bedroom?" he asked. "In my bed?"

"Uhh, yes...yes I did," I admitted, reluctantly.

"Why?" he asked, with disgust on his face. He was clearly troubled by the thought of some sick stranger sleeping in his room.

"Well, because your mom and dad told me to," I said matter-of-factly, not wanting him to think I simply stole his room like a common thief.

"Why'd they do that?" he asked, still concerned.

"I, uh, don't know. You'll have to ask them," I said, as if I too was mystified about how this all went down.

His six-year old brother then emerged from another room. It was no later than 6 a.m., I kid you not. The brother didn't appear quite as concerned that a stranger was standing in the doorway of his bathroom. But then again, I hadn't slept in his room.

"Hi," the older one said. "Wanna play a game?"

I pretended not to hear and slipped past, heading toward the bedroom.

But they followed. As I attempted to climb back into bed, the boys approached me with a box of action figures. They wanted to play. They wanted to play right then.

The youngest one asked me to pick between two characters he had chosen for battle. I chose the biggest strongest action figure, one that could surely squash the other, for I was in a surly mood. The six-year old then had me pick between two figures he was holding. Again, I chose the biggest and the most valiant warrior.

The youngest boy then started smashing the two chosen action figures together in a mock fight. My guy was getting his butt whipped good, anyone could see that. Within minutes, I was informed that my guy was now losing five to nothing. (I am sure this was his subtle way of telling me to never sleep in his room again.)

I fared better with the six-year old. With him, my action figure was only losing three to one.

Unfortunately, I am a bad sport and don't like to lose at anything. So I asked the youngest boy if I could see my guy. He obliged. I took out what I then dubbed my "magic finger" and touched my action figure on the head. He asked what that was for. I told him I had just given my guy ten magic points.

He thought about this information long and hard before calling me a "cheater."

I told him it was not cheating, I has simply used my imagination. But his brother came to his defense, saying I'd used "imaginary cheating." He reduced my magic finger points from ten to one, then used his own magic finger to make me lose that point also.

I gave up and decided to take a shower. But before I could get back inside the bathroom, the younger boy was waiting again. With a painful look, he asked, "You're not going to shower in my bathroom are you?"

The lesson here is a simple one. Cancer patients have many tough decisions to make, including decisions about traveling. There are many options out there, including, at times, the option of staying at the home of a friend or a friend of a friend.

But, as the old saying goes, you get what you pay for.

DARTH VADER

Darth Vader sleeps
at the Houston Hampton
in the bed next to mine

His helmet remains on
and his labored breathing
betrays a mounting fear

for tomorrow we fly
to a pink twilight zone
where pain must be endured

But I won't cry out
and awaken Vader
who's weary from our journey

through space and time
and our visit with aliens
in the sad medical building

Darth Vader likes
Mexican food, but not cerveza
He's a great conversationalist

and reads voraciously
devouring Wordsworth
and Lewis like Jedi Knights

But now he battles
sleep apnea, so I tiptoe past
avoiding a good swift kick

Jim Chastain

7

Vomiting

If I were asked to pick one word that best captures the cancer experience, the very spirit and essence of it, I would have to choose the word vomit. And I think most of my family members would pick the same word, or at least one of its gnarly derivatives.

"Why vomit?" you may be asking. There's no disputing that it's a nasty, vulgar word, one that is somewhat taboo to even speak aloud. I mean, unless you're with a teenager or at a state fair, you just don't hear it uttered in public places. For the most part, it's only safe to use the word in the privacy of your own home.

But vomit speaks volumes for me, insofar as cancer is concerned. For you see, my family has experienced a string of bizarre vomiting incidents since I was first diagnosed. Getting sick has become part of our normal routine, like brushing our teeth, laughing at fundamentalists, and arguing in the car.

Not surprisingly, these vomiting incidents seem to coincide with my trips to Houston for treatment and checkups. Something about these joyous occasions simply makes us hurl.

As I write this, on the evening before I head to Houston for my latest checkup, my temperature is hovering at 101. My son Ford also has fever and one of the worst coughs I've ever heard. How long will it be before one of us begins vomiting? It's almost inevitable.

My daughter Madison, who hardly ever gets sick, has thrown up twice on the night before I was scheduled to leave town for Houston. It's like her little going away present for dear old Dad—the sympathy pains of a distraught daughter—"Here, Dad. A little something to remember me by...blah!"

On one occasion, Madison did her dirty business inside my car, the same one I was driving to Houston the following morning. LeAnn was taking her home from swimming practice, and Madison had one of those, "I'm not feeling good" moments, followed quickly by projectile vomiting.

After it was over, LeAnn attempted a quick clean-up job, but gave up about the same time she started dry heaving. When I went to check how bad the after-effects were, I realized LeAnn's heart just hadn't been in her work. And so I was the one who had the pleasure of spending an hour or so on my hands and knees with soap, scrub brush, and disinfectant.

A seven hour drive is bad enough without, well, you know...that smell. I was determined to get rid of it. And my efforts eventually paid off—I was finally able to make the car smell only slightly nauseating, an acceptable level of funk that I would get used to after an hour or so.

But I guess I shouldn't gripe. I've had my own memorable vomiting experiences.

You see, I'm probably the world's biggest lightweight when it comes to medicine. If the label says, "may cause nausea," I'm guaranteed to lose my lunch. If there are warnings about the possibility of drowsiness, I inevitably find myself in a Rip Van Winkle state of unconsciousness.

And I've had particularly strong reactions to anesthesia. Even with the standard Jim Chastain "pediatric dose," I usually throw-up violently for hours on end.

After my second cancer-related surgery, I didn't even make it to my hospital room before the hurling commenced. I had spent several hours in the recovery room following surgery, drifting in and out of consciousness, waiting for a room to become available. Finally, a great big dude arrived to wheel me to my private room, in my not-so-private stretcher.

"Take it slow," I warned, with a deadly serious tone. "I throw-up."

Perhaps my words were too vague. Perhaps he simply didn't hear me or pay close enough attention, as I was obviously whacked out on painkillers at the time. Perhaps he had a different definition of "slow" than I did. Or perhaps he was a NASCAR fan.

Whatever the reason, he took off at a fairly quick pace and never looked back. We seemed to be flying for a while, as he wheeled me, via stretcher, around sharp corners and down long hallways. The passing breeze was exhilarating, and I felt as though I was on a strange, nausea-inducing roller coaster ride heading straight for hell.

"Almost there," he mumbled.

I seem to remember those same words were uttered by members of one of those doomed Everest expeditions.

If it hadn't been for the elevator, we might have made it. But apparently my body just wasn't ready to leave base camp yet.

I don't claim to know much. But I do know this—you can't put a vomiting guy like me in motion and then come to an abrupt halt inside a steamy elevator.

But that's what the big dude did. He wheeled me into the elevator, and others quickly crowded around us. The air inside was already hot and stagnant, but with all the new bodies on board the temperature soared. From hallway to elevator, the temperature must have climbed twenty degrees.

I started sweating, which is, for me, a sure sign of trouble.

Within seconds, I was feeling sick. An awful tide of nausea began building inside, and there was nothing I could do about it. I was a weary gladiator locked inside a small coliseum with ten spectators waiting to see how long I would last.

You know the feeling...it was no longer a question of *if* I was going to throw up, it was a question of *when*.

I tried my best to fight it. But like an aging boxer, I didn't have it in me.

So I changed tactics. My new goal was to make it a few feet outside of the elevator, for the sheer sake of retaining a smidgeon of dignity.

I think my attendant noticed the green tint that had suddenly appeared on my face, because we shot out of the elevator like a cannon ball. The sudden breeze was helpful to a certain extent, but only in the sense of delaying the inevitable. It was too little, too late.

I saw my room ahead. The nurses were inside, getting it ready for me.

Fifty feet, forty feet, thirty feet. Maybe, just maybe, I could make it inside... But then we hit a small bump in the hallway, otherwise known as the last straw.

As I crossed the threshold into my lovely new room, I began vomiting with gusto. It was like my personal Technicolor announcement to the staff—"Yes, I have arrived!"

The unattractive nurses, who had been smiling, were giving me pained expressions that seemed to be questioning their decisions to go to nursing school. They sighed and commenced clean-up operations. And their work didn't stop there. I gave them plenty more to do over the next twelve hours.

But our most intriguing vomiting story happened on the night before LeAnn and I headed to M.D. Anderson for the very first time, just after my original cancer diagnosis. We were going for a second opinion, to see what the experts at M.D. Anderson proposed to do about my arm.

I can't begin to describe the amount of stress and worry we were experiencing during this time. It was considerable—trust me. I could hardly even sleep. Cancer takes a tremendous toll on you emotionally, and insomnia is a big part of it. If lucky, I would get three or four hours of restless sleep at night, no matter how exhausted I was. And LeAnn was getting about the same amount.

Unbeknownst to me, LeAnn had phoned her gynecologist two days before and ordered a prescription for a well-known (and perfectly safe, I think) sleeping medication. She'd been instructed to take a pill just before going to bed, apparently because it was potent enough to knock her out quickly.

That night, however, LeAnn took her pill, but stayed up a little longer than she should have. She hadn't quite finished packing for our big, stressful trip the next day.

I didn't know she had taken a pill or that she even had a prescription. I was busy packing, watching television, getting ready for bed, wondering if I was going to die.

At some point, I walked into the bathroom and saw her standing in front of the mirror. She was swaying back and forth like a drunken frat boy, clumsily attempting to brush her teeth.

"Are you okay?" I asked, thinking she must be having some sort of stress-related epileptic seizure.

"I tuk a shleeping pill and it... umm, meshed me up up... bad, meshed..." She was slurring her words like the good old girl I knew back in college.

"You have sleeping pills?" I asked. "Why wasn't I invited?"

The joke passed right by her, as if she wasn't even there. And she wasn't really—she was a zombie, the walking dead. A stream of toothpaste was dripping out of her mouth and down her chin, spilling white drool all about the floor and counter.

LeAnn didn't seem to notice. She was concentrating on standing.

I began laughing, my typical reaction to anything so out of the ordinary freaky.

"You'd better go lie down," I advised. "Before you hurt yourself."

LeAnn dropped her toothbrush right there on the spot, stumbled past me, bumped into the bathroom door, and then headed straight for bed.

I began brushing my teeth at this point, shaking my head and chuckling all the while. I couldn't believe how messed up she was. I made a mental note to go check on her in a second, just to make sure she was okay. And then to go get the video camera.

At this point, I heard LeAnn trying to set the alarm. This normally takes about two seconds, but now it went on and on and on. Beep, bing, beep, beep, beep, beep, bing, bing, beeeeeeeeeep.

She's wasted! I thought, as I stopped brushing and headed in to help.

Beep, beep, beeeep, bing, beep. She was trying her best to figure out the alarm clock, which was proving itself a formidable opponent.

"Here, here, I'll do that," I said.

Looking relieved, LeAnn sort of fell back over onto the bed as if she'd just been shot. I set the alarm and then looked at her with amusement. Uh-oh. Her face was white as a ghost and her upper lip was, well, sweaty.

"Are you okay?" I asked, as tenderly as I could in my *oh my god I've got cancer* state.

"I'm uh, not, uh, feeling sho gud," she mumbled. Then her eyes focused on a point on the ceiling, and she got an urgent look on her face.

I know this look. It's the one my kids give me when they're about to throw-up and have no way of getting to the bathroom in time.

I did what I instinctively do when my children get the look. I cupped my hands under LeAnn's mouth, just as a stream of vomit burst from her. My hands filled up so quickly, all I could do was empty them into the fold of the shirt I was wearing, and then hold them out again. Then, she yacked once or twice more.

At this point, she abruptly passed out, with vomit all over her face, her pajamas, the sheets, and, of course, me. Within seconds, she was even snoring a bit.

I carefully made my way back to the bathroom, dumped the contents of my shirt in the toilet, and began washing my disgusting hands in the sink. I took off my soiled shirt and set it down carefully on what would soon become the "contaminated area" of our bathroom floor.

Then I went in to help LeAnn. I undressed her and threw her rank pajamas onto the contaminated pile. Then I sort of rolled her around the bed as I took off the sheets and blankets. I got a warm wash cloth and a little soap and cleaned her up as best I could (there's only so much you can do). Then I went and threw the pile of soiled laundry into the washing machine.

I dressed LeAnn in new pajamas, and replaced the sheets and blankets. She never stirred a bit throughout the whole ordeal as I maneuvered her.

Eventually, I went to take a shower. I remember standing in front of the bathroom mirror and laughing about what had just happened. It started with a chuckle, but before long I was laughing with everything I had.

I mean, there I was, on one of the most stressful nights of my life—before I would head into the unknown, when I would finally talk to someone who knew something about my cancer—and I was literally up to my ears in vomit. Not from one of my kids, mind you, but from my wife! And she wasn't even officially sick—this was self-induced.

But that's life, isn't it, this strange combination of wonderful, painful, and everything in between?

Life doesn't stop when you get cancer; it keeps rolling right along. Despite all the emotional turmoil and horror, you still have responsibilities. You still have to do the laundry, take out the trash, and help the kids with homework.

Sometimes you even have to cup your hands so your wife can blow chow in them.

For better or worse, I once vowed. And for some strange reason, this was part of the better.

MOVIE STAR

When he was a kid, Joaquin starred
in his own action/adventure film.
He was the hero, of course, and saved
many fair maidens and city folk
from dragons and dangerous monsters.
He could fly then and had other
magical powers too, although
he forgot what they were long ago.

As he grew older and went off
to college, Joaquin was in a string
of teenage comedies, *Animal House*
rip-offs, complete with drunken
frat guys, togas, late night burrito trips,
and unmentionable things.
He was the life of the party
in his Belushi-style altered state.

But comedies can grow tiresome,
so Joaquin switched to romance.
He was the dashing leading man
with the woman he loved on his arm.
They had a Tracy and Hepburn, no,
make that Cary Grant and Irene Dunne
type of relationship. A love story
with elements of broad comedy too—
a romantic comedy. The bottom line
was two people finding each other
and living happily ever after.

Since then, Joaquin's mixed it up.
He was in a Grisham-style legal thriller
that audiences hated, some worthy
kids' films, and an ill-conceived drama
about a corrupt insurance company.
He began a religious epic, but bowed out
when the cast and crew quarreled.
His indie about a film critic's trials
and tribulations was seen as too "insider,"
so he did a horror film about an alien
that invades and consumes its victims.
But horror has a limited audience
so Joaquin looked elsewhere.

He went to Broadway and starred
in a Shakespearean tragedy,
but the reviews were mixed
and the play closed after a short run.
He took a minor role in a satire
about some writers who never write,
but just sit around talking about it.
That role revived his career,
and many scripts came his way.

Joaquin now had his choice of genres.
He thought long and hard about
the projects in which he'd taken part.
What sort of role suited him best?
Realizing he was a romantic at heart,
he steered in that direction, for although
he now had less hair and more wrinkles,
one is never too old for love.

8

Bad News

In movies, patients are always alone when they receive bad news from their doctors. That's just the way it is.

The doctor enters the room and says, "Mr. Alexander, your test results are back." Notice the grim look on the doctor's face. He didn't go to medical school to be the bearer of bad news. "I came to help people, damn it!" his face seems to say.

Mr. Alexander, detecting a serious tone and demeanor from his physician, asks nervously, "Is something wrong, doc? I'm going to be okay, aren't I?"

"Well...I'm afraid you have (dramatic pause and drum roll) cancer," the doctor reports straightforwardly, although saddened by the pain he casually dispenses like Pez.

"Cancer? Gee whiz. That's kinda bad. Is there anything you can do?" the patient asks naively, not knowing the Grim Reaper has been following him around like a bad reputation.

"Nope. It's inoperable. You only have six weeks to live," the doctor says, after making some quick calculations. Placing his hand on Mr. Alexander's now-trembling shoulder, the doctors then offers apologetically, "I'm sorry. It's a tough break."

Strangely enough, that is pretty much the way things happen in real life. At least that's been my experience—minus the "six weeks to live" part. (To date, I've managed to avoid hearing those ominous words; however, the word ominous has been used, so there you go.) You have a brief one-on-one encounter with a doctor, who may or may not be a people person, and moments later you walk away shaking, wishing you could recall the doctor's exact words.

I've now received bad news four times, and each time I received it alone. There was no one to witness what went down, no one to take notes, no familiar shoulder to cry on. It was just the doctor and me.

You can look at this in one of two ways. On the positive side, I was spared the indignity of having my tears become a spectator sport. Sometimes crying feels pretty darn good, and I've done my share of it. But as a general rule tears are rarely something you want to share with others. Unless, of course, you're Ben Affleck, who cries in virtually every movie he's in.

On the negative side, there's hardly a lonelier moment in the world than the moment when your doctor announces such devastating news. It's the perfect time for a good old bear hug, so long as you have the right bear by your side.

For me, the first round of "bad news" was a complete shocker, as unexpected as the ending to *The Sixth Sense*. (Yeah, yeah, you were one of the one's who figured it out, right?)

I had simply taken my MRI reports to a local orthopedic surgeon, a month or so after a radiologist had looked at the same images and declared there was less than one half of one percent chance that the minute growth on my right triceps muscle was cancerous (See Chapter 1).

But I had decided to have the darn thing biopsied, just to be sure. Even if the growth wasn't cancerous, who wants to walk around with a lump on their arm? That's just gross! So my MRI images and I went searching for an orthopedic surgeon. We would have the growth removed, confirm that I was A-OK, and then get on with life.

The doctor, a referral, entered the room with my MRI images and clipped several to the wall in front of me. As he did, I entered into this aforementioned, way-too-familiar movie scene. Only here, I was suddenly in the leading man's role. And that's bad because I'm a horrible actor.

"Well, young man," he said with abrupt seriousness. "I have to tell you, I don't like the looks of this. Not one bit. And here's why...see these little fingers here?" (He was pointing to little areas where my "anomaly" seemed to be branching off, or spreading.)

I can't remember much after that. The rest of the conversation is pretty much a blur, except I do remember him putting his hand on my shoulder and saying some well-intended mantra of encouragement. He was a good man who really seemed to care.

I walked out of his office building a few minutes later to a bright, sunny day and a dark, murky perspective. In a moment's notice, my life had changed. My physical health, indeed my very future, was suddenly very up-in-the-air. I could easily become one of those guys in the movies with just six weeks to go.

After a brief Ben Affleck moment of misty-eyed confusion, I morphed into a Woody Allen hypochondriac, one who asked himself question after question without ever pausing for reflection. What do I say to my wife? And my kids. Who would tell them? *Should* we tell them? What about my mom and dad? How would they take it? They had already lost one child, my sister Karyn, eight years earlier.

I called LeAnn from my cell phone. She was in a car filled with women, and they were laughing and having a great time. (You know, no guys around.) She asked, nonchalantly, how everything went.

I replied, "not good."

"What do you mean?" she asked, with more focused concentration.

"He thinks there's a problem. I think he was preparing me for bad news."

This was met with a long silence. Sometimes, there's nothing to say.

We probably managed a few more words, but if we did I can't remember what they were—perhaps something about the MRI and not dwelling on mere possibilities, no matter how scary the situation seemed at that particular time. We tried our best to cling to some vague sense of hope. But six weeks later the next round of bad news would cut much deeper and leave a more noticeable scar.

A lot had happened during those six weeks. I'd had the strange growth removed in an outpatient surgery. We'd been told there was "concern." It wasn't "necessarily" cancer. It could be this or that, although some of the other possibilities were more frightening than cancer. The sample had been shipped around the country from one expert to another, finally winding up at the Armed Forces Institute of Pathology in Bethesda, Maryland. We had entered into an extended waiting period, an excruciating delay of several weeks that took a serious toll on our emotions and physical well-being. Truth be known, we were completely stressed out.

And then it happened. I was at work, trying to keep my mind focused on a case that had been dying on my desk from lack of attention like an unwatered house plant, when the phone rang. I answered it on the first ring. That's what you do when you're waiting for important news about your impending death.

As I heard my doctor's voice, my heartbeat sped to about four times its normal pace. The phone call was brief, and the message was grave. Yes, it was cancer. Not only cancer, but stage three out of four, meaning an aggressive, fast-growing version. He would need to see me in his office. Then he said, "I'm sorry," and we hung up.

Once again, I was all alone when the news hit. Unbelievably alone. It was as if the real world had been swallowed, and I was stuck inside a horrible dream with no means of escape.

Sitting there at my desk in my little office, I felt a strange sensation of terror and relief. I was thankful the waiting game was finally over, but I was haunted by the fact that this was not a game at all. It was a fight for survival. My new job was to try, as best as I could, to hold on.

I stood, walked over, and closed the door. Then I cried. Not hard, but softly and quietly. Gentle Ben Affleck tears for an audience of one.

Then it was time to be a man again and make the phone calls. First, LeAnn. When I told her that same malignant diagnosis, she spoke kind, encouraging words to me. *She is the strong one*, I thought. And she is, although this was surely one of her toughest challenges.

After that, I had to call my Mom and relive the same nightmare over again. But at least here was some payback for all those times she'd made me go to youth choir when I was a teenager.

Needless to say, after these first two experiences, I was becoming a little gun shy about the prospect of being alone when it was time to receive news about my health. There seemed to be some sort of jinx at work, and I was growing scared of being alone when a doctor announced my prognosis.

The way I figured, if I could just keep someone with me at all times, perhaps I could break the spell that had likely been cast upon me by some undercover witch I once dated. If bad news only comes when one is alone, then I would never be alone again.

But it's really not all that easy to keep some handy person beside you at all times, a tagalong who waits with you for news, good or bad. People tend to want to live their own lives, strangely enough. Plus, they don't really enjoy hanging out that much with someone who appears to be, well, more than a little paranoid about their health.

This is surely one of the biggest post-cancer battles of all, trying to keep a healthy balance between paranoia and blind neglect. The goal, I think, is to achieve a state of stable vigilance, one that is attentive to the clear signals the body is sending yet still able to function in society in a fairly normal way, i.e., to have a good day. But it's a hard balance to find, and I've been known to take a tumble or two along the way.

Case in point. About a year later, after I'd had a second surgery (this time at M.D. Anderson in Houston), I found a small knot on the bottom of my arm in the same approximate area that my last tumor had been. Although it was much less pronounced than the first go around and was in all likelihood scar tissue, I was concerned. Anything "new" in my arm was not good.

And so, I found myself walking around and feeling my arm all the time. Often, I would be doing it without even thinking. It drove my wife crazy—the way I would have my left hand twisting around inside my right shirt sleeve, searching around for the Jimmy Hoffa in my arm. And when people spoke to me, I had a hard time concentrating or carrying on normal conversation. I was preoccupied, fighting a battle of emotions and fear that was invisible to the naked eye.

Wild thoughts entered my mind. I had dodged a bullet the first time, by finding the cancer early and having it removed. Could I really be so lucky again? Perhaps the cancer was back and attempting another hostile takeover. My active imagination was working against me as I considered the possibilities.

The general consensus among those closest to me seemed to be that I was worrying too much, perhaps even being a bit obsessive/compulsive about my condition. My prognosis was good, supposedly at the top of the list of those who should survive the cancer. So when I would confess my mounting anxiety about this new place on my arm that may or may not be scar tissue, people would give me a skeptical "he's losing it" look. It's basically the same look people make when watching a Michael Jackson interview.

At some point, I could no longer ignore this new area in my arm. So to calm my fears, I proactively scheduled an MRI in Norman, rather than wait for my next appointment in Houston, which was a month away. But the MRI only revealed "post-surgical changes" that were, most likely, scar tissue. My friends and family had been right. It was just scar tissue, and I was losing my mind. Nevertheless, I continued living by a "be afraid, be very afraid" motto.

A month later, when it was time to return to Houston, LeAnn opted to stay home so she could work and attempt to keep things running smoothly with our kids. I reluctantly agreed that this was the best decision, for it was. But the little boy inside me wished we could have worked it out so she could come.

That way I could avoid the jinx or curse put on me by you-know-who.

My friend John had some business in Houston, so he offered to drive with me. This didn't necessarily mean I would have someone sitting beside me when my test results came in (an ultra-sound, chest CT scan, and doctor's appointment), but at least I would have someone to talk to on the drive.

The morning of my tests, John and I parted ways, as he had to take care of some business. I drove to M.D. Anderson alone, trying my best to remain as calm and collected as possible. I had my chest scan, and then headed to do the ultra-sound, extremely grateful that I wouldn't have to suffer through another MRI.

My last ultrasound experience had been during our second pregnancy, so I pretty much knew what to expect. The technician turned on the monitor, placed some clear gooey gel on my arm, and began searching. Before he got very far, I cut right to the chase. I pointed to the curious spot on my arm and said, "Check right here."

He did, and I was suddenly staring at an ultrasound image of an oval shape inside my arm. I was pregnant! So that was why the MRI tech had suddenly become so quiet...

The MRI tech began measuring things, saving images, fidgeting about in his seat. Then, he excused himself so he could "show this to the doctor." His concern spoke volumes.

As I was waiting, alone again, I shook my head and considered how difficult life can be. I had little doubt the cancer had returned, but still your mind does its best to convince you otherwise. (Slightly more than one year later, I would be in the same room, having the same awful experience again and receiving the same bad news once more.) But whatever it was, I knew I wouldn't hear the "official" news until I spoke to my doctor the next day.

A doctor entered with an extremely long needle, which she began thrusting repeatedly into my arm, hoping to get some "tissue samples." The next twenty minutes or so were some of the most torturous and loneliest points of my life, despite the fact I had three or four medical professionals devoting full attention to my well-being. You don't have to be alone to feel alone.

The next day, John came with me to my doctor's appointment. He was there for moral support, although he seemed to believe my arm was just fine.

Before long, a nurse called my name, and it was time to hear the bad news. As I approached, the nurse asked if I wanted to bring my friend in with me or go it alone.

I paused for just a moment, as I thought how silly my "jinx" idea had been. Whatever news was waiting for me in there, good or bad, it wasn't going to change based upon whether or not I was by myself or with company.

The question was whether I wanted to hear the news alone or with company. Did I want that brief moment of privacy—the chance to grieve if bad news came my way? Or did I want someone there to give me the bear hug?

"No, I think I want to do this on my own," I said.

I still have no idea if that was the right answer.

REGARDING FRODO

How strange when we identify
with fictional characters
to this degree

I'm no Tolkien freak
but I've discovered
a hobbit camaraderie

by wearing a burdensome ring
that taunts and burns
and consumes my energy

The fellowship would help
bear it but there's only
so much they can do

as I tiptoe alone
along Mordor's borders
where Black Riders wait

Someday I hope to be free
of the curse and drop
the damned thing in the fire

to put on my real smile
and relax once more
with my Samwise friends

9

MRI

I have this *slight* tendency to get claustrophobic.

It has little to do with small spaces really. I can crawl through a narrow tunnel, no sweat. I can hide inside a broom closet during a game of hide-and-seek with my kids without negative repercussions. I drove a Nissan Sentra for years and never had a single problem.

But when I'm in a small space and can't move, that's when I start getting nervous. Especially if there are ventilation issues.

Elevators are a good example. I could easily ride to the top of the Sears Tower with five or so people on board. But increase that number to fifteen people and turn off the air conditioning and my skin starts to crawl.

I gotta have room to move, air to breathe. So in that sense, I'm a bit claustrophobic.

This minor phobia may have something to do with my second year of college. I was living in a fraternity then and, as stupid frat guys do, I joined nine pledge brothers in a wrestling match with three brutal seniors—huge hairy guys who lived to punish freshmen and sophomores.

We were holding our own for a while, so long as we kept a three-to-one advantage. But then a couple more seniors decided to join the party. The tide quickly turned. Before long, four or five separate matches had become one great big Wrestlemania mass, like a swarm of snakes in a farm pond.

My goal was to stay at the edge and top of the pile. Some deep sense of survival told me to keep away from the middle or bottom; that, or I didn't want the muffled cries of anguish coming from deep within to be my own.

But then someone caught me by the leg and started pulling me into the swarm. No matter how hard I tried, I could not escape. The massive pile of sweaty arms, torsos, and legs engulfed me, and I was quickly pushed to the bottom. And there, I found my head pinned against a concrete wall.

I knew right away that I was in serious trouble. I couldn't move. My head was about to be squashed by the sheer weight of the idiots encircling me. This was not unlike one of those human stampedes that takes place every now and then after a European soccer match or rock concert, leaving fifteen or so people trampled to death.

My life passed before my eyes. I would never see another beautiful sunset. I would never find and marry that special girl. I would never go to another keg party.

I had to do something...

My only out was to start yelling. So I YELLED as LOUD as I possibly could!

But no one heard me. They were all too busy kicking each other's butts.

I had no alternative but to let out the best high-pitched, blood-curdling girl scream I had in me. You know, the kind you hear in horror movies when an unsuspecting co-ed discovers she's about to become the next victim. I gave it all I had.

Thankfully, the girl scream worked. Someone near the top of the heap said, "Hey, there's a chick down there." So everyone slowly untangled themselves from the pile, to see how a girl got in the mix and whether or not she was good looking.

I was free! I would live! I would drink more beer!

"Never again," I vowed. I would never allow myself to be trapped like that again.

And I wouldn't—at least not for another eighteen years, when I would enter the MRI tube.

MRIs have been a regular part of my cancer maintenance. With my particular cancer, a form of sarcoma, recurrence is a primary concern. That being so, MRIs are used to detect areas in my arm that I can't see or feel. I generally have an MRI every six months or so, unless my doctor extends grace and opts for the less-demanding ultrasound.

For those of you who don't know, during an MRI you must lie deathly still with your entire body inside a narrow tube for about forty-five minutes, listening to a series of surging pings and metallic beeps. (You often get to listen to music on headphones, but not always.) In the end, the MRI technician gets a picture of the inside of your body that resembles an x-ray or ultrasound, only with more detail.

Of course, MRIs are an absolute nightmare for people who are claustrophobic. Sort of like mountain-climbing for someone with vertigo.

But for someone like me, one who is only slightly claustrophobic, MRIs aren't all that bad. Although they can be...

About six months after having two surgeries to remove the cancer from my arm, I went back to the hospital for my much dreaded six-month checkup. With cancer checkups, each time you go is the "big one," for the odds of recurrence decrease with each visit. But the six-month checkups are particularly important, because that is when you have the most tests done. I have a whole battery of tests, including blood work, an x-ray, a CT scan, a manual check by my doctor, and, last but not least, the dreaded MRI.

The six-month cancer checkup is kind of like being the frog in biology class, minus the smell of formaldehyde. You are continuously poked and prodded and ogled. It's a long, exhausting, nerve-wracking experience. And my first six month checkup proved to be especially nerve-wracking, one of the worst ordeals of my cancer experiences.

The fun began with me standing in a line of cancer patients, as one so often has to do in cancer land. (Cancer hospitals are like Disney World, minus the rides, ambiance, and joy.) We were waiting to have IVs put in, because, with many MRIs, one has iodine injected in order to get an enhanced image.

I was sitting beside an older man who was probably seventy or so. He seemed to be deep in thought or, worse, discouraged.

This was one of those moments cancer patients experience time and time again—the opportunity to engage or not engage the person sitting beside you. I had to choose between staying quiet in my own little world, or being friendly, sharing the whole cancer experience with those around me like one shares the common cold.

On this particular occasion, I decided to talk to the man.

"So, what ya in for?" I asked, in mock-convict speak.

"Leukemia," he answered, matter-of-factly.

"Oh really. How long have you known?"

"Couple of weeks," he said. "I was feeling kind of run-down, so I went to see my doc in Pampa. He did some blood work and then, bang, he drops the bomb."

"So...what's the prognosis?"

"According to my doc, two or three months."

"Wow," I said, in my eloquent way. One hardly knows what to say in these situations, but "wow" seemed to cover it.

"Yeah," he replied. "I asked him what my options were, and he told me to get my things in order. I said, 'That's it?' And he said, 'Hey, this is what happens when you're seventy-four.' I didn't like that answer, so I came here."

This was a new perspective for me. As a thirty-eight year old husband and father of two, I had received a different response from the medical community. Cancer was not supposed to happen to me. I was "so young." This was a "bad break" and so forth. With me, the doctors spoke of being aggressive and vigilant, not passive and accepting.

How sad, I thought. At some point in time, if we live long enough, our reward may be a "Well, what did you expect?" attitude from the medical community.

Our names were called, and my friend and I were escorted to the tiny IV room. Unfortunately, I drew a newcomer on her "first week." (By the way, these are words you never want to hear in a medical setting, especially when the speaker is holding a big needle. Trust me.)

To make matters worse, I am one of those people with "small veins." Small veins are not an asset when someone is trying to insert a needle into you. Whenever IVs are an issue, you want to have the biggest freaking veins possible.

In cancer land, small veins and a novice assistant are collectively known as a "bad combination."

The novice commenced the procedure with a pat, pat, pat on the back of my hand.

"Okay little vein...come out, come out, wherever you are," she said, in a Big Bad Wolf voice.

After two unsuccessful tries and a bit of spilled blood, the now extremely-nervous assistant called for reinforcements from the hospital's "IV expert," a little Asian woman who was widely recognized as an intravenous miracle worker.

A woman sitting across from me said the Asian woman was the best. "I have small veins too," she revealed. "I always ask for her."

"Thanks," I said, to my small-veined friend.

But just as the miracle worker began heading my way, the door opened and in walked one of the largest human beings I had ever seen. He was a young man who must have weighed, I kid you not, 600 pounds. I think he had glandular cancer or something.

Three or four tired and frustrated workers accompanied the man. They'd been unable, for obvious reasons, to locate their subject's veins. After fifteen or so misses, they had come seeking help from the miracle worker.

"Happens every damn time," he said angrily. "You people can't ever find my veins." As if this was somehow their fault. Needles and haystacks, you know.

Anyway, his appearance was bad news for me. I was bumped for a "bigger priority."

The novice assistant took this news hard. She was still shaken by my recent blood loss. But she faced her fear and found my vein on the next try. I let out a huge sigh of relief and smiled. "There, that wasn't so bad," she offered in a shaky voice, with sweat pouring from her forehead.

And it wasn't so bad, when you put things into proper perspective. Sure the needle missed twice and I lost a little blood. But by comparison, I had suffered little. That guy over there was practically a pin cushion, or perhaps some sort of cursed voodoo doll.

That's the thing about time spent in a cancer hospital. Whenever you start feeling sorry for yourself, there's usually some poor soul close by who will make you feel like the luckiest person on earth.

And so, my friends and I—the elderly man with leukemia, the small-veined woman, and the jittery assistant—watched in captive horror as the miracle worker began searching for her new patient's vein...in his neck.

"I'll never complain about an IV again," I promised.

At this point, my name was called. They were ready for my MRI. I left my new friends there in that little room. They may still be there, for all I know.

I've come to discover, through my experiences, that MRIs weren't designed with arms in mind. Under normal circumstances—assuming there are "normal" MRI circumstances—you really aren't all that cramped during an MRI. You lie in the middle of the tube unencumbered, except for the IV in your arm. Under this setup, you have approximately twelve inches between your head and the top of the tube, and at least another foot of free space on either side of you.

That's plenty of room to move around. Plenty of air to breathe.

But arms are tricky. To accurately measure one's arm, the arm must be positioned as close to the center of the tube as possible. For me, this means lying on my back with my left shoulder pressed firmly against one side of the MRI tube. Meanwhile, a foam pad is placed between my right arm and chest, to separate the two, and my arm is then strapped down in a way that is virtually unmovable.

And remember, I have this slight tendency to get claustrophobic.

The trick, of course, is to remain calm and regulate your breathing. If you can do that, you'll be okay. MRIs usually last about 45 minutes. That's a long time to remain calm, but it's do-able, especially with the help of Valium.

And so, after receiving the obligatory ear plugs (for lessening the surging, pinging noises), my MRI nightmare began.

I was lying inside the tube, trying my best to take my mind off where I was, what they were looking for, and how bad it would be if they found something. I hadn't eaten all day—you can't eat on the day you have an MRI—and so I started thinking about food. Maybe LeAnn and I would eat at P.F. Changs that night...

I actually drifted off for a few minutes.

Sometime later, a loud voice from some hidden-away speaker woke me: "This next one will be four minutes, Mr. Chastain."

This meant that the next series of metallic pings and surges would soon begin and would last about four minutes. I'm not exactly sure how MRIs work, but I do know that the machine takes different readings that last anywhere from one to ten minutes.

To pass the time, I tried counting the minutes, because, well, I tend to count things. And soon, I'd estimated that I was halfway done. Then I drifted off once more.

"This one will be seven minutes, Mr. Chastain. After that, just one more and then we'll do the iodine."

My arm was starting to ache. It was positioned awkwardly, and a past shoulder surgery I'd had wasn't making things any easier. My arm was throbbing, but I could take it. *I'm a man,* I told myself, unconvincingly.

After seven minutes passed, a five minute series started, supposedly the last one before iodine. I was almost finished. "Good," I thought, because I had to pee.

"This next one is four minutes, Mr. Chastain. Then just a couple more."

What was that? Did he say we were going to do another one, AND THEN TWO MORE? I must have misheard him.

After the four minute test ended, we launched right into the next test without any sort of warning as to how long it would be. I began counting, trying my best to stay calm. But my breathing had quickened, and I could feel my heart pounding.

The unusually long test finally ended, but then a new one began without warning.

What was going on here? Was something wrong? Why was I suddenly so hot?

My internal alarm clock told me I was already well past the hour mark, and we hadn't even introduced the iodine yet.

The test finally ended. But then A NEW ONE BEGAN!! Ping, bing, bong. Then the sustained surging noise, uhhhh, uhhhh, uhhhh, uhhh. Approximately ten minutes.

Why all the additional tests? Maybe they'd found something new growing in my arm. Perhaps I was in trouble again. Perhaps the cancer had returned. This would mean surgery, bills, pain, grief.

Sweat began pouring down my forehead like rain in a gutter. My arm was aching, and my left fingers were tingling, meaning I was losing circulation from it being pressed against the wall for so long. I hadn't had to pee this badly since college.

The next test ended, and then ANOTHER ONE BEGAN!

OH MY GOD! I thought. Another test? I would never make it. I started freaking out. What in the world was happening? I'd been in there for an hour and a half.

I hit the panic button.

Most MRI machines have a button that a patient can hit to inform the technicians that something's wrong. I pressed mine repeatedly.

"Yes?" a calm voice said, like HAL, the computer in *2001: A Space Odyssey*.

"What the hell's going on out there?" I asked. "I was supposed to be out of here thirty minutes ago. Is something wrong?"

Pause and then a weak, evasive, "No."

Uh-oh.

"We're almost there, Mr. Chastain. Just a couple more," he told me, as if I'd lost all ability to count.

"You've already told me that two or three times."

"We're trying to get some better shots."

"My arm's cramping, and the other one's falling asleep. Plus, I have to pee."

"Can you hold it?" he asked, as if I were five.

"I'm not sure," I said, wanting to make him as nervous as he had made me.

"Well, let's finish up this one, and we'll get you out of there."

As we completed this last test, I had time to think about his words. What did he mean by "some better shots?" Had he found something, but needed to look at it more closely? Maybe he just screwed up the first batch and had to get some more.

I was suddenly cheering for my MRI technician to be lousy at his job. That seemed better than the thought of him taking a closer look at a particular area in my arm.

When they finally pulled me out of there, I hobbled over to the bathroom, like an old woman carrying a bucket of water. I took care of business, then headed straight to the MRI technician.

"You found something, didn't you?"

The technician exchanged a startled glance with the person working beside him. They had a rogue cancer patient on their hands.

"I, uh, really can't talk about results, Mr. Chastain. It's against hospital policy."

"I'm not asking you to give me a diagnosis. I'm just asking if there was something you were particularly concerned about."

Another quick glance at his friend. An odd, evasive look.

"I'm sorry. I can't talk about that."

He was clearly lying, the way his eyes were shifting back and forth. I was reading him like a cheap novel.

He assisted me back to the MRI tube, where I endured two more scans and then two more after the dye was injected. My heart was pounding hard as I thought about what had happened, about each word he had said, each look, each shift of his eyes.

Maybe I was just being paranoid. Maybe he just screwed the first series up. Maybe he had seen something in there, but it was just scar tissue. But his eyes. It was hard to dismiss his eyes.

I finally decided it could go either way. I had no hard proof that my cancer had returned. All I had was circumstantial evidence.

When they finally pulled me out of the tube, I was a physical and emotional wreck. I'd been inside for more than two hours, which had to be some kind of record, and I had nearly lost my mind along the way.

LeAnn met me as I left the room.

"Where have you been? What took so long?" she asked, not angrily, but with concern.

"I think they found something. They kept doing more and more tests. It was a nightmare." I was on the verge of a complete breakdown.

My wife held me tenderly, and it was just what I needed. Human touch can heal in ways that even medicine cannot.

We had a quiet dinner that night, trying our best not to think about my doctor's appointment the next day, when I would learn the official MRI results. We had been at this place many times before, the waiting place. It wasn't getting any easier, only more familiar. You certainly couldn't dwell on it.

The next day, I learned my MRI results showed no recurrence, only what appeared to be scar tissue. I'd nearly lost my mind worrying, but everything was under control, at least for now.

Cancer is every bit as much of a mental and emotional battle as it is a physical one. You are never really "cured" for the condition lives on in your mind and nightmares. Each check-up presents the very real possibility of bad news, of a new battle, of additional heartbreak. Sometimes you've got to give it all you got just to keep from going crazy.

And sometimes you lose the battle.

An MRI presents special challenges, for in there you are alone with your fears. On this particular occasion, those fears defeated me, resulting in my own version of cabin fever, a combination of isolation, paranoia, building anxiety, and bad memories.

Not to mention the fact that I have this slight tendency to get claustrophobic.

POEM THAT HAS NOTHING TO DO WITH CANCER

10

GOD

During my cancer journey, I haven't always had the time or energy or desire to try and figure out "what it all means." The physical side of cancer can be demanding and exhausting. But the spiritual side of cancer, that is the philosophical and theological side, is often overwhelming.

But a cancer patient can't simply ignore cancer's spiritual implications. For as maddening as it all is, cancer is, by and large, a spiritual journey. Cancer forces those of us who have been diagnosed to closely examine what we believe about God, healing, miracles, faith, and the meaning of life—apart from anyone's well-intended words or religious clichés.

During the last three years, I've hardly spent a moment apart from the word cancer. Like that Willie Nelson song, cancer is "always on my mind." It's as much a part of me as my bad knee, love of movies, and silly hair. The "c" word follows me like a shadow. Sometimes long and ominous, three times larger than I am in real life. At other times, it's small and barely noticeable, but there all the same.

I suppose no single word has occupied more of my mind and thoughts in the last few years than that frightening word. But the word "God" may be close.

"Cancer" and "God" are words/concepts that go hand-in-hand. They are forced partners, Siamese twins joined at the hip. Like peanut butter and jelly or Sonny and Cher. One word leads to the other, and vice versa.

Cancer...God...

Cancer/God

Cancer: God.

Cancer? God!

People diagnosed with cancer will inevitably think about God all the time. Some must face, for the first time in their lives, the question of whether God is out there at all. For those who make it past that significant hurdle, never a given, there are other questions waiting. Who is God? Why did God let this happen to me? Did I do something wrong? Does God really love me?

Or perhaps this is one of those book of Job bargains with the Devil. Am I just a lab rat in a cosmic experiment? (If so, how do I get off the spinning wheel?)

And then you get to the more practical questions. Will God heal me? Does prayer help? Is this part of "God's plan for my life?" Have I been chosen to suffer? How do I find that highly touted "peace that passes all understanding?"

Cancer! God?

In August of 2001—just after I'd had a biopsy performed on the tiny bump in my arm—the surgeon who had performed my operation called to tell me the radiology department was "concerned." Although the mass they had removed wasn't "necessarily" cancer, the doctor began preparing me for bad news. In so doing, he gave me the medical names of three possible conditions I might have, two of which were forms of cancer.

What does one do with information like that, having the bare names of three possible medical conditions without knowing anything more about them? Sit on the information and cross your fingers? Put it out of your mind and dwell on positive things? Pray the whole thing will just go away?

Perhaps.

But that's not what I, the modern man, did. For I had the internet waiting to tell me everything I ever wanted to know. Or at least thought I wanted to know.

That's right. I made the regrettable mistake of surfing the internet that night. And the end-result was one of the darkest moments of my thirty-something life.

Make no mistake, I'm not advocating ignorance here, i.e., adopting an "I don't want to know" approach to health. I've read several books where the authors have encouraged patients to be their own doctors, to do the necessary research to learn everything possible about their conditions, for doctors are certainly not infallible. I think that is an honorable approach, and probably the wisest (and toughest) one to follow. However, internet research has its own particular dangers. The information may be old, it may be written in a confusing manner, or it may not even be accurate. There is as much chaff as there is wheat when you're conducting internet research, and that is difficult when your research is a matter of life or death.

I started my research by typing in the name of the form of cancer my doctor said was the most-likely candidate, malignant fibrous hystiocytoma (MFH). Within a few seconds, I was directed to a site that addressed that condition in great detail. I remember reading in horror that the treatment for MFH consisted of immediate amputation of the entire arm, including the shoulder. Also, the site was kind enough to inform me I had about a 33% chance of surviving one year.

As it turned out, this was bad information. Part of it was my own fault, for the statistics were referring to MFH of the bone, not the muscle tissue. But I had no idea at the time that there was a difference between the two. All I knew was the condition was affecting my arm, and so I naturally concluded these statistics were applicable.

A dark cloud descended over our bedroom when I read these statistics and then relayed them to LeAnn. We fell into a somber *Oh my God* state of existence. I was 37 years old, mind you, with two young kids. It was a horrifying moment in our lives, one that words will never be able to adequately describe. Of all the dark moments we have experienced—and there have been many—this was probably the darkest.

I headed for the shower, where I do my best thinking, and started sorting through the horrible possibilities. I was going to die a painful death. My kids would grow up without me. My parents would lose their second child. LeAnn would move on. She would remarry in the standard one to two years. A new husband would move into my home and raise my kids. Ford would throw the baseball with his new dad. Madison would have someone else walk her down the aisle. I would be, at some point, forgotten.

I was freaking out, having been confronted with the very real possibility of becoming a fading memory.

When I went to bed that night, my heart was racing as never before. It felt as though my heart would explode right there in my chest cavity.

I'd heard of panic attacks, but until that night I thought they were reserved for hypochondriacs and octogenarians, usually female. But I've since come to know, first hand, that panic attacks are very real, for I was in the process of having one.

My mind turned to God. Being raised in the Christian faith, I'd been taught that "God is my refuge and strength, a present help in times of trouble." And so, I tried my best to pray to God that night, to plead for my life and for my family. But I couldn't concentrate. I was so overwhelmed by grief and fear—a state of sheer panic—that it was hard to even form a complete thought in my mind.

Despite my best attempts to access strength and peace from God that night, I failed miserably. I hardly slept at all. I was like Atlas, with the weight of the world resting on his shoulders. But in my case, that weight was centered on my chest.

The next morning, I got out of bed and tried to think of something to do. What do you do when confronted with the fact that your life is literally on the line? You certainly don't turn on the TV, I can promise you that.

I picked up my Bible, for I was in desperate need of some answers, or at least a bit of comfort. God was still out there, I told myself, despite my inability to find peace. I flipped through the New Testament, trying to decide where was the best place to start reading. I considered pouring over the Easter story, remembering that Jesus had experienced an emotional battle in the Garden of Gethsemane, where he literally begged God to save him from the cross. But, to be honest, I didn't want to read about Jesus' march to face death on that particular morning. While that could conceivably be where my own road was headed, I still hoped this cup might pass.

I turned to the Old Testament book of Psalms, a book filled with honest prayers of grief, pain, fury, and existential questioning from various writers. Here was the place where I might find some comforting words. Or, better yet, where I could find one of those really angry Psalms, where the author rages over God's inexplicable silence.

I landed randomly on Psalm 16 and began reading.

Now I don't believe a person's faith should be built upon randomly selected Bible passages accessed during times of crisis. A "relationship" with God, whatever that means, has to be more intimate than that, much less magical and hocus pocus haphazard. Sure, consistent reading will lead to the discovery of passages that relate to real experiences you are having at a particular moment in your life. But it seems pretty clear to me that God's revelations are not based upon the erratic throws of a finger-pointing dart.

Nevertheless, I've come to believe I experienced one of the true spiritual moments of my life that morning through Psalm 16.

I'll admit it's a paradox—believing you've encountered God in a particular way. We search for a spiritual life, one where God leads us, but then bristle and roll our eyes when someone claims they've "heard from God." We even doubt when something bordering on the supernatural happens to us.

But if God is really out there and was ever going to communicate with me in a more direct way, this was the perfect time. At that particular moment, I was struggling like never before, unable to find words to pray in the midst of my grief and sorrow.

Is it possible that God took pity upon me and was moved by my tears? I later learned that my wife had seen me reaching for my Bible and had immediately prayed that God would communicate with me that day and give me comfort and guidance. Perhaps God answered her prayer and recognized that I needed direct intervention, an encounter that was more personal than I'd ever before experienced. (Or perhaps I'm in need of serious psychiatric assistance.)

Anyway, the first two lines of Psalm 16 immediately grabbed my attention: "Keep me safe, O God, for in you I take refuge. Apart from you I have no good thing."

What a great prayer for one who has been overwhelmed by a flood of cancer-induced emotions. Here were the simple words I could not utter or find the night before. "Keep me safe, O God, for in you I take refuge. Keep me safe, O God. Keep me safe."

In the following weeks, I would pray this prayer over and over, at those times when my mind could think of nothing else to say. Indeed, I still pray it quite often, for my battle with cancer is far from over.

And then, in verses five and six, Psalm 16 says, "Lord, you have assigned me my portion and my cup; you have made my lot secure. The boundary lines have fallen for me in pleasant places, surely I have a delightful inheritance."

These words reminded me how much I'm blessed, apart from cancer. Along with some significant challenges, God had given me an abundant portion: a wonderful wife, two beautiful, healthy, and talented children, a supportive extended family, one of the best groups of friends in the world, a good job, a nice home in a free country, and access to quality medical care. The boundary lines had indeed fallen favorably for me—I had a delightful inheritance. I still do.

I pondered the words, "you have made my lot secure." Was this a reference to the writer's physical possessions and family or his final destiny? Perhaps both. And could they somehow apply to me? I surely longed for that to be true.

Such theology could be debated forever—whether God uses words that are thousands of years old to communicate with us today. I completely respect those who believe the answer is no. But I was comforted by the idea of my lot being secure. Whether that was a reference to the present or the future, it was still good stuff to hear. My lot needed to be secure.

I read on.

Verses seven and eight sent chills down my spine. And they still do today, as I write these words more than two years later: "I will praise the Lord, who counsels me; even at night my heart instructs me. I have set the Lord always before me. Because he is at my right hand, I will not be shaken."

I have already told you how my heart had been shaken on the previous night. Here, however, the words reminded me of God's presence throughout the night. For me, this would come, primarily, through the prayer I had already committed to memory. "Keep me safe, O Lord, for in you I take refuge." These words, I vowed, would be a useful reminder that God is a safety net when I am falling.

But verse eight was the grabber. The Psalmist "set the Lord always before" him, allowing God to pave his way. And there was no reason to be shaken, for God remained close to the Psalmist, at his "*right hand!*"

Need I remind you that the cancer was in my right arm? That I was at that very moment facing the real possibility of having my right arm amputated, which, of course, would include my right hand—the hand I used for writing, typing, throwing the ball to my son, and holding my wife and daughter's hands?

For obvious reasons, it felt very good to consider God being at my right hand, no matter what the outcome.

I had rarely experienced any Bible passage that applied so directly to my situation. The applications were piling up so high it was becoming difficult to explain them away as sheer coincidence.

In verses 9 and 10, Psalm 16 states, "My heart is glad and my tongue rejoices; my body also will rest secure, because you will not abandon me to the grave, nor will you let your Holy One see decay."

Now I understood the eternal implication of these words. While I'm not exactly a "Holy One," as a Christian I do believe my spirit will live on after I die, in heaven, a better place. So in that sense, it was wholly consistent with my belief system that I would not be abandoned to the grave or see decay.

But again, as one who was wondering, *at that particular time,* whether or not I was about to die, the words "my body also will rest secure" had a more personal meaning. Was this some sort of personal encouragement? Were these words an indication that I was going to make it through this cancer ordeal and live to tell about it?

I don't know, quite frankly. As I write this, two years later—after suffering through four surgeries and two recurrences of cancer—I'm still wondering whether or not I will make it, whether my arm will be amputated, whether cancer will spread to my lungs, whether or not those horrible things I thought about in the shower that day will eventually come to pass.

So, although I'm not taking the position that God gave me a "promise" of healing, I can tell you this: on that day in August, more than two years ago, I felt strongly I had experienced God in a very real way. Call me crazy, but I came to believe God had wanted me to know that things would turn out okay. That I would live to tell my story.

So that is what I am doing right now. I am telling you my story, my testimony. What happens from here, God only knows. At some point, we will all eventually die.

But I'm doing my best to faithfully believe I will survive cancer, that I will beat it. I remain hopeful, or perhaps "cautiously optimistic."

Yet that doesn't mean I never experience fear. I often wonder whether my time for resting secure is coming to an end. But I have to put those thoughts aside if I have any hope of enjoying the life I have today, right now.

In the meantime, Psalm 16 is my rallying cry. In the last verses, David says that God has "made known to me the path of life" and that joy has been the result. I feel like this is at least partially true for me. The road to joy has often been rocky. I have seen the highest of highs and the lowest of lows. At times, I have been completely overwhelmed by grief, and my faith has been sorely tested. But overall my life with cancer has been somehow richer and more real than it was before.

Still, I keep praying.

Keep me safe, O God, for in you I take refuge.

Keep me safe, O God.

Keep me safe...

Amen.

FAMILY

four will be
three
three will be
two
two will be
one

three bury
one
two bury
two
one buries
three

cruel world where
four
can't just be
four
and always be
four

11

Lower Extremities

I opened my eyes and saw blurry shapes.

I was in bed, but not at home. It was dark, but only because the curtains were pulled. A nearby TV emitted the familiar sounds of a football game, but without my glasses, I couldn't tell who was playing. Someone was sitting close, leaning toward me.

It was LeAnn. She was smiling.

"Surgery's over. Your doctor took out the tumor and said it was very small. But she found another spot and had to take another centimeter around that too. She had to sew your triceps back together. The doctors tested the margins, and they were good."

Bittersweet words. I'd made it through this, my third cancer surgery on my arm, but there were additional signs of spreading. My mind, although under the effects of anesthesia, still knew this was not great news.

LeAnn looked tired, but was still able to put on her brave smiling face.

I drifted back to sleep...

Thirsty.

I awoke again, but was still very groggy. And this time, there was both thirst and pain. I noticed a bandage on my arm with strange tubes sticking out of it. Oh yes, the radiation tubes, for later. Who knew they would be so big?

My shoulder wasn't hurting this time. That was good. I remembered how much my shoulder had hurt after my last surgery, because my arm had been held in an awkward position during the operation.

"Just press this button here, if you have pain," LeAnn said.

I pressed the button.

LeAnn slid my glasses onto my face. My vision returned. I focused on the television, as if out of instinct. Oklahoma State versus Nebraska. And OSU was...winning. This must be one of those dreams within a dream.

I noticed a slight pressure on my bladder. I would have to stand soon and go to the bathroom. This would mean vomiting. Oh well. It was to be expected. That's what I do.

I closed my eyes again and nodded off...

My eyes opened. More awake this time, I looked at my tiny room. LeAnn was reading. She looked up and smiled again.

"Hi. How are you feeling?"

"Okay. Is that OSU?"

"Yeah. They're about to beat Nebraska."

I started calculating the odds. They were astronomical. OSU had never beaten Nebraska in football during my lifetime. (Thirty-eight years!) It was much more likely that I would die of cancer within the year than there was of an OSU victory. But here they were, winning. For some reason, that didn't make me feel too good.

"I have to pee," I said.

"I, uh, think you still have your catheter in."

One thing a male patient is never told before surgery is that as soon as he is sedated, he is stripped completely naked and a catheter is inserted into his penis. I imagine "catheter inserter" must be one of the worst jobs in the world, on the same level as cleaning out a liposuction machine or clearing a minefield.

I decided I should take a peek, just to see what a catheter really looks like. After all, I had only heard of them before. During my previous surgeries, they had always been removed before I ever knew they had been there.

Using my good arm (while LeAnn was not watching), I maneuvered my hospital gown around until I could get what is referred to in Southeast Oklahoma as a "look-see."

Ugh. There it was all right. The dreaded catheter tube, piercing me through.

This wasn't exactly a Kodak moment. I felt, somehow, like a fish on a spear, a Mer-Man of sorts, the "catch of the day."

Plus, I felt so...violated. Who had done this to me? Every person in the hospital who smiled at me from this point forward would be a suspect.

So...if I have a catheter in, why do I need to pee? I asked myself. Perhaps I should have asked the nurse this question, but I was afraid that, if I did, she might want to make sure everything was all right down there. That wasn't going to happen. There was no freaking way!

I would just have to grin and bear it. Be a tough guy. I mean, think of all the men who had been prisoners of war during World War II. Surely I could endure this irritating bit of pressure upon my bladder.

Besides, by the look of that disgusting bag at the end of the catheter tube, it was pretty clear I was urinating quite well. Indeed, I could see the pee flowing upward in the tube. Now how was that possible? I surmised the process must be similar to siphoning gas from a car. Unfortunately, this reminded me of how the siphoning process begins, which was...extremely troubling.

As the day passed, the anesthesia within me began to slowly wear off, and I was able to stay awake for several hours at a time. I chatted with LeAnn and my nurses, as if nothing was wrong. But all the while, the nagging feeling that I needed to pee continued. To tell you the truth, it was starting to drive me a little bit crazy, like some sort of heinous Chinese water torture.

At some point, my torment became too great, and I began asking questions. One of the nurses was kind enough to explain that the tube put pressure on my bladder and made me feel like I needed to pee, when I really didn't. It's basically the same feeling a woman has in the late stages of pregnancy, when her belly balloons to the point that it puts constant pressure on her bladder.

In addition to these long overdue sympathy pains, I had the added bonus, during my mandatory afternoon "get out of bed" walk, of experiencing what it's like to be one of those guys who has had his prostate removed and, as a result, carries a stylish urine bag around on his hip. Some guys carry a gun on their hip. Others carry keys and a beeper. For me, it was a fashionable bag of pee.

Anyhow, as the day of surgery was drawing to an end, I was still in agony. Despite the noble efforts of the vigilant nurses who kept coming into my room and emptying disgusting bag after disgusting bag, I never got the comforting relief one feels whenever leaving the toilet after a job well done. And it was driving me crazy.

To make matters worse, new catheter issues emerged during the night. Issues that will require some amount of delicacy.

It has been my experience over the years that men often awake in the middle of the night, more toward morning really, with—oh how shall I put this—a boner. This isn't, necessarily, a sexual thing. It seems to have more to do with gravity and a full bladder, although one never really knows about those things. But it happens frequently and there doesn't seem to be anything a guy can do to prevent it.

On this particular night, I awoke in my hospital bed at about 4:30 a.m. or so. And I was like...WHOA! WHAT IN THE WORLD IS HAPPENING TO ME?

Without getting too graphic, let me just say that a catheter is bad enough without, well you know, but it is pretty much unbearable in that particular state. (One thing is for sure: I'll never be able to eat another corndog.)

In hopes of curing my condition, I tried to relax and concentrate on something that was so thoroughly nauseating and disgusting that it would somehow reverse the process. I imagined my anesthesiologist entering the room with a big hairy booger hanging from his nose. This seemed to help. I recalled recent terrorist attacks. Much better. Choir music. Yes! That toenail on my dad's foot. Oh yeah! I was on the road to recovery.

Now, in a much-improved state, I looked at the TV, which we had left on for a bit of noise during the night. A sexy commercial was on.

Uh-oh.

The next day, at the crack of dawn, I began asking when I could have the catheter removed. The nurses were evasive. They were unsure how long I needed to keep it in. It was the weekend, and doctors were scarce.

I became a total pest to every nurse or staff person who entered my room that day. No matter how difficult it was to turn the conversation to catheters, I somehow managed it. At some point, I began begging them to make the catheter go away.

They would respond with a patronizing smile. But finally, one of my nurses let the cat out of the bag, so to speak, and told me someone would be in to remove the catheter "soon."

Soon is one of those vague words that can mean different things to different people, depending on the situation at hand. To me, soon meant ten minutes or less. To the nurse, however, soon meant whenever the "catheter person" got around to it.

During the hour or so between my version of soon and my nurse's version, I had time to contemplate the magnitude of what was about to happen to me. Someone was about to enter my room, and pull a tube out of my penis. Surely they would send in a man, wouldn't they? But then again, that would be pretty weird and probably not all that gentle. Gentleness was a must as far as I was concerned.

My heart began beating fast.

Enter a small African American female nurse, approximately twenty years old.

Oh my God!

"Are you ready to have your catheter removed, Mr. Chastain?"

"Uh-huh." Damn. My voice had cracked, like I was a sophomore in high school.

"I, uh, think I'll step out for a second," LeAnn said. I didn't protest. There are some things a man has to do on his own.

As soon as my wife left, the little nurse went right to business. She had me sit on the bed with my legs dangling over, and she rolled up my hospital gown to mid thigh. I now looked like I was wearing a very bad mini dress. But at least she hadn't yanked the entire gown off, leaving me there in all my nakedness.

The nurse donned gloves. This was good. Very good. I wasn't exactly sure how things were going to go down, but at least I wouldn't have to deal with cold hands.

She reached under my gown, as if she were a doctor and I was about to give birth. Her hands glided up the plastic tube until they rested at the very end of my, er, enis-pay.

"Okay. Get ready. You're going to feel a sort of tug, and then a dull pain."

How does one "get ready" for a tug and pain? No one had offered me a bullet to bite. Catherine Zeta-Jones hadn't entered the room to hold my hand and tell me, "You can do it, stud." And so, I simply smiled and said, "Let her rip," which, in hindsight and by the odd look the nurse gave me, was about the worst thing I could have possibly said.

It is impossible to describe what it feels like to have something pulled from you, something that is attached to your insides like the cord of a lawnmower. It was a strange sensation, that I can remember, and it lasted longer than I thought it would. There was a sharp pain, at first, but in about five seconds, the misery had ended and I was free from my bondage.

The nurse left me alone with my blushing cheeks and sore wiener.

LeAnn returned. "So?" she asked.

I started crying.

Not really.

I probably said something to show how tough I was, something like, "Piece of cake" or "catheter, schmatheter." But all I can remember saying was, "I gotta pee."

Man, I felt old.

I entered the tiny bathroom and shut the door behind me. Still wobbly on my legs and aching from my middle, I decided to sit down and pee, girl-style. This was the safer route. People frequently died in bathroom accidents, for goodness sakes. Nobody wants to go out like Elvis.

I assumed the position and waited for what I thought was going to be the most satisfying urination episode in my life.

But there was a problem. Some sort of gurgling began bubbling deep inside me, as if my pipes had a clog or something. I concentrated harder.

And then I had the weirdest experience of my life: my penis let out what amounted to a fifteen second long fart, followed by a series of shorter farts that sort of burped their way out.

It began slowly—like a sputter. But then, after the first muffled gasp, a sustained burst of energy came from me, as if I had been consuming pork and beans for the last week. It tickled like all get out. Plus, my unit began bouncing around wildly, as if someone had just turned a rolled-up water hose on full-blast.

As the fart continued, I began laughing uncontrollably. And then, with each additional new blast, I laughed even harder.

"What are you laughing at?" LeAnn asked from outside.

"My penis is...farting!" I guffawed.

"Huh-uh," she said.

"Swear to God," I replied.

This is what cancer had reduced me to—a pathetic man with fifteen tubes hanging out of my arm. A small girl half my age had just violated me. I was wearing a rolled up gown, sitting on a toilet like a girl, and farting from my penis.

Whatever dignity I had left that day in that hospital bathroom. And yet, it all seemed very funny. Life is crazy. Hospitals are crazy. And catheters are crazier still.

TUSKS

Many elephants
were lurking about
that cold Thanksgiving day

but nobody dared
to talk about them
and risk being trampled

How surprising then
to discover that I was
the biggest elephant of all

The circus was
in full progress and
my tusks were showing

12

Left Behind

The supreme happiness of life is the conviction that we are loved;
loved for one's own sake—let us say rather, loved in spite of one's self.
—from *Les Miserables*, by Victor Hugo

The cancer had returned. It was rediscovered during one of my quarterly
checkups at M.D. Anderson, and I was scheduled for surgery—my
third, if you include the original biopsy—in October of 2002.

LeAnn and I prepared for a five-day stay in Houston. After all, this was
how long my last surgery and recovery had taken there. Why should this
time be any different?

On the first day, I was scheduled to meet with a radiation oncologist
and then have an MRI, to locate exactly where the cancer in my arm was
now lurking. On the second day, I would see my regular doctor and have
blood work done. On day three, I would arrive at the hospital before sun-
rise, and the cutting would commence. After recuperating in the hospital
for a couple of days, I would head home, where my precious kids would
be waiting.

Five or perhaps six days, at most, then home for the holidays. Or so
we thought.

I wasn't exactly sure why I'd been asked to consult with a radiation oncologist. I'd already been through six weeks of radiation therapy in Oklahoma City, and it had been ineffective. The cancer had returned in less

than a year and seemed to be laughing at those feeble efforts. And that was supposedly all the radiation my arm would tolerate. But perhaps some new innovative radiation technique had been discovered during the last year, like some sort of localized device or laser blast during surgery. I mean, there had to be a new option available, or I wouldn't be going for a visit.

"It's called brachytherapy," the oncologist explained. By my best guess, he was five years younger than I was, perhaps thirty-five years old. But that was fine. I was beginning to get used to this new paradigm, being older than the superhero doctors who were determined to save me.

"You see, after your doctor removes the mass, we insert tiny catheter tubes through your arm in the area of your incision, where the cancer was removed. Then, you heal in the hospital for three days. At that point, we feed a radioactive wire into each tube. You'll be radioactive and stay isolated in a room for about four days. Then, we'll take out the wires and tubes, and you go home."

Piece of cake.

I had so many questions my mind couldn't begin to process them all. How "tiny" were these tubes? Would they hurt? What did he mean by "isolated?" Isn't it slightly dangerous to be radioactive? What did this mean for my future? Would my brain be fried? Would I grow a third nipple?

And was there any available empirical data that this treatment would help me?

"Listen, your cancer has already proven it's resistant. After your first surgery and radiation, you had about a ninety percent chance that the tumor would not return. But it has. So we know this is a nasty dude. With surgery alone, you probably have about a fifty percent chance that the cancer will return. But with brachytherapy, we hope to increase the chances to seventy or seventy-five percent."

Always with the percentages. My life was constantly being estimated and measured. Health-wise, I was like a developing hurricane, and this oncologist was the meteorologist studying me from a safe distance.

"But I've already had radiation," I reminded him, just in case he hadn't checked my progress notes.

"Yes, but this is better. Brachytherapy is more localized. The catheters run through your incision. It's a low dose of radiation, but constant, right on the most dangerous area. It should kill any remaining bad cells without further damaging your arm."

I paused.

"It's your best option," he said. "It's what I would do."

And so, with those words, I agreed to the procedure. Then we broke out a bottle of post-consultation champagne.

Okay. Not really.

What a kink this brachytherapy threw into our plans. We had only worked out childcare for five days. Now, I was looking at being gone for at least a week and a half, if everything went well.

And the last days would be spent alone in an isolated room.

"There's no way I'm going to go home and just leave you," LeAnn said, in her matter-of-fact way. "I can't do that."

But what were our options? In a regular hospital room, LeAnn could stay with me, sleeping on one of those little chairs that makes out into a decent cot. But during my time in isolation, she would have to check into a hotel room. This would be costly, and she would have to miss work. Not only that, visitors to the isolation unit could only stay for fifteen minutes a day, standing across the room behind a lead shield.

Having her stay in a local hotel didn't seem like a sound financial decision. Plus, we had the kids to consider. How would they respond to us both being gone for so long?

"There's really no choice. You have to go home," I said, using my most noble tone of voice, totally faked. "We can talk on the phone everyday, as much as we want."

So another hard decision was made. LeAnn would go home to be with our kids and get in some work. I would become a Wal-Mart bestseller: *Left Behind.*

It was a tough call, and LeAnn was struggling with it. These were emotional times for us, and we were hanging by tenuous threads. Perhaps she was unsure how well I would hold up, for I'd had been fighting depression. Plus, it wasn't in LeAnn's makeup to leave when there were responsibilities at hand. It was in her blood to "stand by her man." (In a wholly unthreatening, non-fundamental sort of way, of course.)

The day she left was like one of those sad goodbyes soldiers have when heading off to war. It was a pretty melodramatic scene, and I remember it vividly.

Four days after surgery, I could get around the hospital fairly well. I drew a few stares, of course, walking around in my pathetic hospital gown and pajama bottoms with my arm in a sling and fifteen catheter tubes extending awkwardly from the sling. But so what? About 20% of the people you see walking around M.D. Anderson look like they could collapse and die at any moment, and another 20% look like they're already dead. *Compared to them,* I told myself, *I'm the cream of the cancer crop!*

LeAnn and I walked outside, hand in hand. We hugged. We said a few words. We cried. Then she kissed me, turned around, and walked toward the parking lot. It was like the ending of *Casablanca*, only I, Humphrey Bogart, didn't have Claude Rains waiting for me when she, Ingrid Bergman, left the runway. Plus she stopped to chat with someone she knew, thereby robbing me of the opportunity to watch her walk out of view. After a few minutes waiting for her to stop talking, I said "oh, what the hell" and headed to my room in the isolation wing.

It was a spacious and luxurious room, for a hospital. I had a remote control bed and a large TV with cable, including one channel that showed first run movies all day long, like pay-per-view without the pay. (I'm sure it figured into my hospital bill somewhere.) I had a VCR, and a long list of movies from which to choose. I had a comfy chair. And I had a big bathroom with a shower that was custom-designed for a guy who wanted to keep water off his arm.

The hospital's menu had just about every food imaginable—tilapia, shrimp, smoothies, French fries, omelets, coconut crème pie, chicken cordon bleu. I could order anything from the menu whenever I wanted and as often as I wanted, no charge. (I'm sure it figured into my hospital bill somewhere.) I was like a convict having his last meal, three times a day!

I also had a long window that extended completely across the north wall of my room. If I sat in the windowsill, I could see downtown Houston. *This will be a great place for journaling or reading the six books I brought,* I thought. My isolation would, at least, give me time for the contemplative life.

I wasn't exactly roughing it. But, hey, what can I say? Those people at M.D. Anderson...they sure know how to do cancer.

There was only one problem: my room also came equipped with a big lead door that was custom designed to stay tightly shut. So, no matter how great the perks (and they were great), this was still a self-imposed jail cell.

And then, complications arose. During her seven hour trip home, LeAnn had driven into a torrential downpour. The windshield wipers on the car we'd borrowed had stopped working, and, unbelievably, the windshield itself had come loose from the molding that held it in. LeAnn had managed to tape the windshield down, and the wipers had started working again, just barely. But she didn't know if she should risk going further with the car in that condition. I checked the Weather Channel and told her it looked as though she would soon be in the clear. She opted to plod forward.

I slept fitfully that first night—a combination of LeAnn's scary journey home and the anticipation of radioactive wires being inserted in the morning. The road ahead was uncertain, and my sleep patterns were letting me know it.

My radiation oncologist and several others arrived bright and early with medical equipment in hand. They would do the procedure in my room. I met a new member of the team—a novice who would be doing his "first brachy" (with my radiation oncologist supervising, of course).

Oh joy.

It's never great to hear you've been given a first-timer, so I was less than thrilled when I discovered the novice, Brad, would be handling the procedure. While the thought of making a personal contribution to the field of medicine sounds nice, when push came to shove I couldn't care less about that crap. I wanted expert hands inserting those wires!

Things didn't go well.

The problem was "catheter number three." Unfortunately, it was sitting against my nerve. Thus, every slight movement Brad made to the catheter caused pain to shoot through me, and my arm would flinch spasmodically in response. Sort of like testing the reflexes on your knee, only with considerable pain.

I imagine Brad was one of those guys who had always caused the buzzer to go off when playing the childhood game Operation. As he clumsily fed a radioactive wire through catheter number three, he managed to repeatedly jerk on the tube and reengage my nerve. I, in turn, was doing my best not to scream my famous girl scream (see Chapter 9). But I couldn't control my body language: balled-up fists, a tightened jaw, pained grimaces, tears streaming from my eyes, and clenched buttocks.

There was a thick tension in the air. One of those in attendance actually had to hold my other hand so I wouldn't jump up from the bed.

"Ahhhh!" I finally gasped, through gritted teeth.

"Does that hurt?" Brad asked with a poker face. He was apparently not one to rely solely on outbursts of agony. He needed corroboration.

I think I said something kind like, "Hell yeah!" My Baptist upbringing was beginning to give way, or perhaps shine through.

Upon hearing my profanity, the team leader came to the rescue. "We're going to need a local and a sedative," he told a nurse, who hurried from the room. A couple of shots and two pills later, I was feeling better. The procedure continued, and Brad, now looking rather gun shy, continued slowly inserting the radioactive wire with his ever-shaking Janet Reno hands.

After catheter number three was completed, the worst of it was over, although catheter number four was also near the nerve and caused some tense moments. The remaining wires went in smoothly, like a foot sliding into a comfortable old shoe. Meanwhile, I crashed from the stress and radiation and the sudden inflow of drugs into my system, the best sleep I would have during my four day stay in isolation.

I awoke in my room hours later. I was alone.

My time in the isolation room was strange. It wasn't so terribly bad in the beginning, but by day four it was torture. It was the loneliest I've ever felt in my life.

It wasn't that I didn't have human contact. I did. A maid entered my room once a day and hurriedly changed my linens and left new towels. (Add this to the list of world's worst jobs.) The room service people would drop my food by and then get the heck out of there. A nurse who probably drew the shortest straw checked my vital signs once a day.

I received phone call after phone call from well-meaning friends and family, on average about ten a day. And every night ended with LeAnn's voice, which helped me make it to morning. I also received several gifts and care packets, including numerous gifts and cards from my wife and a gag package from my work friends that included a can of Spam, a douche, a Jesus light, and an aluminum radioactivity hat.

But brief, forced contact with a stranger or two is no substitute for meaningful community with those you love. Talking on the phone is no substitute for face-to-face conversation. And gifts and cards cannot replace human touch. I missed seeing my wife and getting bedtime hugs from my kids.

Plus, there was way too much time to think. Most of the time, my busy life kept me from dwelling on all the cancer possibilities. But in the isolation room, I had all the time in the world to think about where I was and what I was facing. As a result, a sense of melancholy began to spread over me like the plague.

Anticipating something like this might happen, I had brought my journal along so I could write my way out of the misery. Unfortunately, my arm, loaded down as it was with tubes and radioactive wires, made writing difficult. I couldn't find a comfortable writing position, plus I had no energy. The radiation was like Kryptonite sapping my superhuman strength.

So I read and ate. I talked on the phone and watched movies. I slept, but not well. I watched construction workers in the rain on top of a building across the street. I took long, cautious showers. And I stared at the hands of the clock across the room as they moved slowly around and around. I counted the hours and minutes remaining and thought of home.

On the third day, I had my first visitor, a friend of a friend. I'd never met him before. He arrived out of the blue and told me he too was a "cancer survivor" who'd spent time in isolation. He had a jagged scar across his nearly shaved head from some cancer-related surgery.

He walked past the lead shield and sat on my bed, two immediate no-nos—and then he began telling me his secret for making it through the ordeal: his "hope hoop," a bracelet he'd made out of a hemp-like rope.

"Whenever I got really down, I'd just look at my hope hoop," he said. "And I'd say, 'I can do this. I know I can do this.' And then I would perk right up."

I smiled and waited for the punch line. When I realized it wasn't coming, I began searching around for the hospital remote, the one that allows you to call for help. Just in case.

My new buddy then handed me a hope hoop he'd made for me as a gift. I accepted it awkwardly, slipping it over my wrist and tightening it according to his instructions. Words were hard to come by. I thought about saying, "When do we smoke it?" or asking if he had some more for my friends on Uranus, but decided against it.

As you may have guessed, I was in no mood to entertain complete strangers. And the thought of placing my hope in a bracelet, even if it was only intended as a symbol, was not working for me. (A year later, the Lance Armstrong yellow bracelet would become a national phenomenon. So I guess he was onto something.)

I mean no disrespect to my visitor. This was a nice gesture from someone who went out of his way to come cheer me. The fact that his offer backfired is no reflection on his heart. His gift was thoughtful and kind, surely worth a crown, or perhaps a bandana, in heaven. Still, it was pretty darn weird.

My parents dropped by a few hours later. Mom brought her camera, of course, and began snapping pictures of me in my pathetic state. "Oh come on, smile!" she actually said. I wondered if one of the photos would wind up in her Christmas card: "And here's one of Jimmy getting the radiation."

Meanwhile, time crept along slowly, like a baby with a loaded diaper. For some strange reason, days in isolation last thirty-four hours, not twenty-four. And time slows down even further if you start worrying about radiation seeping into your brain.

Or so I've heard.

I finally made it to my last night. The doctors were scheduled to arrive at noon the next day to remove the wires and catheters. I would grab a shuttle to the airport, get on a direct flight to Oklahoma City, and do my best to be home by sundown.

My only thoughts were of my family—of LeAnn, Madison, and Ford. In just thirty-four hours, I would see my kids. My wife and I would curl up in our cozy bed and sleep. I'd wrap my arms around her and never let go. "There's no place like home," I chanted over and over, feeling a kinship with Dorothy that was a bit unhealthy for a thirty-eight year old male.

I wrote a poem that night, the only writing I accomplished during my time in the isolation ward. (It's at the end of this chapter.) I had been looking out my window, northward, across Houston, and imagining what it would be like to simply float across the sky and land at home, in a *Waking Life* sort of way. Then I imagined sailing in some sort of magical boat or driving in the fastest of cars or running all the way home. I was actually willing myself there, trying my best to exert the necessary mustard seed of faith to accomplish time travel. But I remained grounded.

I spoke with LeAnn on the phone that night. She'd sent me a Tom Waits CD with a song we love called "I Want You." I listened to the song and longed for home.

We discussed plans for the next day, what time I would be home, when she should pick me up at the airport. We voiced concerns about the removal of the radioactive wires and catheter number three. I would surely get a sedative before the procedure. This would mean it would be a real fight to make it home.

That night, I slept fitfully. I distinctly remember looking at the clock, relieved each time another hour had passed.

When morning officially hit, I showered and packed my belongings. Then the phone rang. It was LeAnn. She asked how my night went. And after I told her, I asked what she was doing.

"Oh, I'm just driving in the rain over by Rice Village," she said. Rice Village is an area we often frequent in Houston. "And I was thinking I might pick us up some lunch from *La Madeleine's.*"

LeAnn had taken an early flight from Oklahoma City that morning to help bring me home. She was in Houston, just a few miles away. It was about the best news I've ever received.

A half hour later, she was standing in my room. She helped me dress after the tubes were removed. She drove me to the airport and helped carry my luggage. She was there to lean on when I started feeling sick at the airport. And she was there to cuddle up next to when I finally made it home.

In the end, it all boils down to those you love, I guess, and those who love you. I don't know if I could have made it through this particular ordeal without the support of my wife, my friends, and my family. My heart aches when I think of those who don't have such a wonderful support system and must do cancer alone.

In certain ways, cancer has been a blessing, for it has constantly reminded me to value those around me with everything I've got. I know it sounds cliché, but we really can't afford to take our loved ones or our time here on earth for granted. Family and friends are precious, irreplaceable gifts. Everything we've accumulated or hope to some day accumulate is meaningless and pales by comparison.

Please trust me on this one. Nobody should *ever* be left behind.

COMING HOME

Sailing
far away from here
in a magic boat
on a silver sea
Cresting
over gentle waves
till I see the land
nestled in my dreams

Flying
with the pillow clouds
under winking stars
in a silent sky
Gliding
with my broken wing
toward a hidden strip
where it's safe to land

Driving
down a lonesome road
in a thunderstorm
without map in hand
Turning
on familiar street
where a handsome house
waits with knowing smile

Running
through a golden field
in the neighborhood
where the foxes play
Hoping
that the bed is warm
and the girl I love
takes me in her arms

13

The Cancer Card

From time to time, we all find ourselves in situations that are difficult and challenging, don't we? Circumstances that are tricky—from a relational point of view.

Someone wants you to do something you'd rather not do, go somewhere you'd rather not go, or spend time with someone you would prefer to avoid at all costs. Someone has plans that will surely take a good chunk of your precious time, plans that inevitably make you feel obligated to participate.

If you "just say no," you risk hurting that person's feelings, damaging your position, or affecting a relationship you treasure—or at least one you need or kind of like. And then, there's the associated guilt...

We face these dilemmas all the time. Aunt Agnes calls about the family reunion just three hundred short miles away. The funeral for your neighbor's grandmother conflicts with a lunch date with a good friend. The office is holding a going away party for someone who is "retiring" (but, of course, there's more to the story). Your son's baseball team is washing cars or, worse, selling beer as a fundraiser. You've been invited to a boring lecture, a couples shower, one of those pyramid scheme parties, an uncomfortable dinner, or a wedding of someone you don't really know.

What you need is a good excuse, one that will help you avoid a miserable time and simultaneously save face with someone who just wouldn't understand why you'd rather skip the event altogether.

"Uncle Bob's gospel quartet is having a lawn concert?...And all the cousins are going to be there?...And watermelon, too?"

This would be a good time to pull out the cancer card.

Membership has its privileges.

Strangely enough, I really do own a cancer card. I use it whenever I go to M.D. Anderson in Houston. It is blue plastic and has my name and a designated patient number on it. (Apparently, I am one of 484,000 or so lucky recipients of this card.) It's kind of like owning a Visa card, only you use it to obtain heart-stopping medical appointments rather than unnecessary merchandise.

But that's not the cancer card to which I am referring. The one I access is a little more vague and not quite so rectangular and plastic.

Now I'm not particularly proud of what I'm going to tell you. And I'm not saying the actions I will be describing are morally right, or noble, or even good for society at large.

But there have been times when I've responded to some of these "come to this event or feel guilty about it" invitations by saying something like, "Gee, that sounds great, but you see, I've got this appointment in Houston..."

Notice this isn't an outright lie (unless you want to get philosophical or legal about lying by omission). My artfully arranged words are technically correct, for I'm always going to Houston about my cancer, at least every third month or so. It's just that, sometimes, I fail to explain, with my carefully chosen phrases, that I'm not going to Houston until two or three days (or, sometimes, weeks) after the crucial event.

Of course, if there's a direct conflict, I throw in all the pertinent, beneficial details. "A potluck supper at the Baptist Church? Gosh, that sounds great, but I'll be in Houston, darn the luck. You know, cancer."

The cancer card is one of the greatest and most effective excuses ever invented, except for the whole "cancer" part of it. Most people simply refuse to challenge it, because they don't really want to know that much about cancer or any of the disgusting details. Just mention the C-word, and people tend to fidget. They get this nervous look in their eyes. They say, "Well, good luck with that" and head toward the nearest exit.

The cancer card works best in church surroundings, where everyone is looking for a good excuse to stay home. (And you'll need a good one, for those folks can spot a bogus excuse from miles away.) It is also useful for excusing one's self from impromptu committee meetings and inconvenient family gatherings. The only exception is when the gathering is for the specific purpose of getting to see you, the cancer victim "who may soon die so we better see him while we still can."

Now I don't want to imply that cancer is the golden ticket to a self-absorbed, "it's all about me" lifestyle. No, no, no. I'm not promoting anything that blatantly narcissistic. It's not about using the card so you can do what you want anytime you want without ever thinking of anyone else. That would be irresponsible, and I've sworn I'm never going to do it again.

But it's important to understand that cancer, quite literally, puts a new light on everything you do. It causes one to take inventory on what's significant in life. Some of the things that once seemed extremely important or at least quite necessary suddenly give the impression of being very beside-the-point, if not entirely stupid.

"You're having a meeting for the Committee that forms Committees? Well, then you'll need to take a look at this handy card I carry."

"You're having a meeting of the Reformed Moderate Democrats who used to be Libertarian Republicans? I'm terribly sorry, but I have this little card that says I never have to do anything that inane ever again."

When you live your life in three month increments, as I do, the thought of wasting three hours at these "keep yourself busy" events seems patently ridiculous, like throwing money in the street. I know it sounds cliché, but time is much too precious for events that merely keep us unbelievably busy.

And so, the cancer card is a useful means of keeping your emotional health intact—of maintaining your sanity in the midst of a silly world and its guilt-induced obligations.

The trick is to only use the card when you really need it, to avoid abusing its wondrous powers.

Plus, the cancer card also comes with two important cautions. First, you must actually have cancer. To fake cancer would be evidence of a serious character flaw that makes you unworthy to be treated in a humane way. Cancer is serious business, and you'd better treat it with respect.

The second caution is this. Unfortunately, the cancer card doesn't last forever. Like a battery, it loses power over time.

Whenever you are first diagnosed, cancer can literally get you out of just about anything, including continuing education courses, tiresome chores (grocery shopping, mowing, and the like), even work.

"You're organizing a neighborhood protest about that nuclear power plant they're building by the elementary school? Sorry can't be there. Cancer."

"The Pastor Search Committee is giving a report? Wish I could, but I've come down with the cancer."

"The birthday party is at Chuck E. Cheese this year? Damn this cancer!"

"A meeting on changes to our insurance coverage? No can do... cancer."

But after awhile, the card is less effective. It only lasts as long as memories do, and people are incredibly forgetful. What once might have gotten you out of driving the Girl Scouts to camp or a work-arranged picnic at the zoo, will eventually only be good for leaving an event fifteen minutes or so early.

And at some point, the cancer card stops working altogether. The expiration date has passed, or people no longer accept that type of card. And then, as with any credit card, you're left with a massive bill to pay.

Someone will comment that *everyone* must pitch in if the committee is going to get anything accomplished, and several eyes will glance your way. The coach will indicate that the team's fundraising efforts are only as good as the "weakest link," followed by a memo showing who he's talking about. A friend will accuse you of somehow letting her down at a time when you were just trying to live.

A relative will complain that you've missed a lot of family gatherings lately and "people have been talking." A business associate will bring up the problem of free-riders. The minister will preach about how it takes a village and the joy of serving others. Someone at work will say you've fallen behind or ask why your work product hasn't been up to its usual standards.

You, in turn, will contemplate being brutally honest. You'll think of saying something like, "Well, I've been having quite a time of it as a result of surgery, radiation treatments, the isolation unit, MRIs, recurrences, mounting financial debts, extreme emotional turmoil, and all the havoc this has caused my family. And I've been seriously questioning the choices I've made in life, the mind-bending monotony of day-to-day existence, my value as a human being, and the meaning of life. To tell you the truth, I've been fairly depressed, unable to work or sleep or eat because I'm concerned about how long I'll live, what will happen to my family, and what legacy I will leave behind."

But you can't say things like that. Not in the real world, which often has very little to do with being real, ironically. No, you just apologize, say you don't know what happened, and promise to do better the next time.

You take your medicine, so to speak, and leave the cancer card in your pocket. Why? Because the card has expired.

It's understandable, I guess. Like it or not, we live in a competitive world where most of our objective value comes from our achievements, the stuff we've put up with and accomplished along the way. Cancer is a tough break—in the beginning—but after awhile it inevitably becomes just another obstacle along your journey. It's certainly not a get out of jail free card.

They may say "take all the time you need" and really mean it. But later, if you are unable to keep up with the pace of life those sentiments will turn into sour grapes. They'll dub you a slacker, eventually forgetting you even had cancer. "Yeah, it seems like he had some health problem at one time or another. What was it? Something like diabetes or hemorrhoids."

That's the way it is. Life has a way of moving forward.

EXCUSE NOTE

To whom it may concern:

Please excuse Joaquin
from the following
until further notice...

> church business meetings
> > committee work of all kinds
> weddings of those he doesn't know
> > political discussions
> office going away parties
> > funeral sermons
> struggling relationships
> > fundraisers
> pyramid get rich schemes
> > summer "event" films
> continuing education seminars
> > anything involving choirs
> home movies
> > malls
> Branson, Missouri
> > school bingo night
> overzealous parents at the game
> > huntin' and fishin'
> meaningless conversation
> > wars

he's got a bad case of the cancer
and doesn't care for such things
and life's too short

> yours truly, Joaquin's mom

14

Timeline

My daughter and I used to play this game when she was little. I would take her hand, during church or some other "stay quiet or else" event, and I would squeeze it four times. This meant, "Do you love me?" Madison would squeeze back three times, meaning, "Yes, I do!" I would then squeeze two times, which meant, "How much?" And she would squeeze my hand once, as hard as she could, showing me the depths of her love by the force of her squeeze.

The game didn't work quite as well when we switched tasks. I was always afraid I'd hurt her hand if I squeezed too hard. Consequently, my squeezes were never quite as hard as she thought they should be in order to show my undying love.

Oh how I miss those days—when my kids weren't embarrassed to take me by the hand, when they would tell me they loved me without hesitation. It's amazing how quickly things change. Moments like that come and go in the blink of an eye.

Time is so precious! I know that sounds corny, but it's one of life's simple truths. And for those of us living with the dark cloud of cancer hanging over our heads, it's somehow even more true. We can actually feel time passing away.

I've been a father for more than a decade, approximately thirteen years as I write these words. And about a quarter of that time has been spent in a dual role, as both a father and a would-be "cancer survivor."

People often tell me they can't imagine what it must be like to have cancer and children, to go through the whole ordeal as a young husband and father. I, in turn, can't imagine what it's been like for my kids. I mean really...what is it like for a young child, not yet a teenager, to find out his or her father has that terrible, dreaded, and mysterious disease? Can their minds even begin to process it?

I wonder...have my kids suffered permanent emotional damage as a result of learning, much too soon, that life is precarious, that one's health can go downhill in an instant? Have their perceptions of me changed to a significant degree? Like the common cold, have my moods affected (or infected) theirs? Has the whole cancer experience offered anything positive, at least in terms of bringing us closer and making them stronger?

I don't know. But I've come to believe that children are all too often the silent victims of cancer. It seems to me that they are the ones who suffer most when cancer strikes a family in the way it did mine, for children are often left to go it alone. Their big questions remain unanswered, as "grown-ups" are busy grieving and struggling to get by.

To be honest, I have few concrete memories of my children, then ages seven and ten, during the first couple of months of my cancer ordeal. This is embarrassing to admit and horrifying to me now, but most of what happened during that period of time has been wiped from my memory banks. Only a few brief glimpses survive.

I remember driving Madison to swimming one day just after we'd received the bad news. As I listened in, she began telling her friends that I had cancer, in a ho-hum matter-of-fact way. That was the first time I had been outed as the "cancer dad," and it hurt. She then went on gabbing with her friends, passing quickly to the next subject, while I was struggling to concentrate as I drove.

Weeks later, I remember being at M.D. Anderson just after my cancer surgery when LeAnn was speaking to Ford on the phone. We'd been away from home for many days, and Ford suddenly asked, "Mom, is Dad dead?" Shocked, LeAnn reassured him I was fine, that I was right by her side in my hospital bed, and that we would be returning home soon. We were puzzled, indeed troubled, by his question, wondering how he'd gotten an idea like that in his head.

But beyond these painful incidents, I remember little. There seems to be a black hole in that place where such memories are stored. Or perhaps it's not that I can't remember, but that there simply are no memories. Perhaps the awful truth is that I spoke very little to my kids about cancer in the early days, simply because the pain of those conversations was too much to bear.

For a while I didn't even know how my kids first found out I had cancer. I assumed LeAnn was involved in telling them, but I wasn't sure. I only knew I wasn't there when they received the official news.

But Ford remembers it, and he recently told me how it happened. "I was in my bed sleeping, and I heard Mom and Madison crying in your bedroom. I got up and asked them what was the matter, and Mom said, 'Your Dad has cancer.' And then we all just sat there on your bed crying."

I suppose it was probably a good thing I wasn't there when LeAnn told the kids the bad news. Judging by how miserably I handled it when we had to tell the kids our beloved dog Daisy had been hit and killed by a car while they were away at camp—I cried harder than the other three put together—it wouldn't have been pretty. If I had been there, they may not have recovered.

Plus, there's a good chance I wouldn't have recovered either, for in the weeks after Ford told me that story, an image of that episode haunted me like a castle ghost. I can close my eyes and see my family there on the bed crying, right now. It is a frightening scene, and I pray that it will never happen again.

The conventional wisdom is that kids are resilient. They supposedly bounce back quickly from all kinds of adversity. At least that's what we're told.

But I often wonder how true that is. Are kids somehow able to deal with tragedy in a positive way that adults cannot? Do they have a built in resistance or a grief-proof soul? I doubt it, for strong evidence keeps trickling in that my cancer impacted our kids significantly, much more so than they ever voiced aloud.

Ford's question—"Is Dad dead?"—shows how easily kids can be left out of the loop of information when cancer strikes. During those days, LeAnn and I were barely making it through each new day's decisions and tears. We spent the better part of our time talking about cancer to doctors, friends, and extended family. So at the end of the day we had little energy (or desire) to try to explain all the details and gruesome possibilities to our kids.

Besides, what would be the point? We didn't actually know what was going to happen. Wouldn't it just be best to leave them in the dark?

But kids inevitably pick up on such things, and parental stress is no exception. Trust me, stress isn't something you can easily hide. It tends to bleed all over the place, like a hemophiliac boxer. When cancer strikes, kids seem to take on that parental stress and add it to their already confused psyche. Eventually that stress begins to reveal itself.

For example, after LeAnn and I returned from one lengthy hospital stay, Ford experienced a clinging period, when he didn't want to be away from us for any significant length of time. Even going to school bothered him. Was this separation anxiety? Fear of losing his dad? Just regular old school day blues? Or something else? I don't know. But I believe his fears were cancer-related.

Madison, on the other hand, seemed ticked off by the whole cancer thing, as if angered that such things are even possible. Whenever my health was mentioned she would say, "You're going to be fine, Dad," in an exasperated tone, never entertaining the possibility of a bad result. That's how some people cope.

But there were other clues that cancer was taking its toll on her.

At school one year, Madison and Ford were both given the same assignment—to do a "timeline" of their lives. Not surprisingly, "Dad got cancer" made both final drafts, as one of the five or six big events. It was something like...vacation to Florida, second vacation to Florida, Dad got cancer, Daisy died (and Dad cried like a baby), got a skateboard for Christmas. The fact that my poor health was at the center of their work product was significant. It doesn't take Freud to figure that one out.

Madison recently shared a poem she'd written during those days called, "Hard Times." The poem says: "Every night I want to cry. Please Dad try not to die! Don't you dare, please see I care. The doc is fair, you'll keep your hair."

That is so Madison, taking a tough issue head-on and mixing in morbid humor along the way. Apparently I'd voiced some concern over losing my hair if chemotherapy wound up being part of my treatment. Madison expressed what she was feeling, then took some of the edge off with a joke. I do the same thing.

Madison also shared an essay she'd written for school called, "I Changed When." In the essay, she tells of staying with her grandmother while I was having surgery in Houston. She wrote, "It was horrible, but we got through it and survived." Brief, but right to the heartbreaking point.

Ford also let his fingers do the talking. He wrote a poem about my declining health, saying, "You'll make it, I'll make it, We'll make it through the hard times in life."

Ford also wrote an essay at school called "What My Father Means to Me," which was entered in the Father of the Year Contest held by the National Centering for Fathering, an organization headed by Ken Canfield in Kansas City.

I didn't even know about the contest. The first time I learned about it was when I received a notice in the mail that Ford's essay had been chosen as a finalist, which meant his essay was in the top 36 out of 1,500 submitted! It also meant that I was suddenly in the running for Oklahoma City's Father of the Year, which was ridiculous, considering how out of it I'd been since my cancer diagnosis.

It's difficult to describe my emotions when I received that notice in the mail and read Ford's essay. There are moments in life, brief moments, when you get a little glimpse of something better, when you feel as though things are going your way. That was one of those moments for me.

Ford's essay spoke of our strong relationship, how I play sports and games with him, read to him, and make jokes "all the time." He also wrote about how I had lived through cancer, saying, "Sometimes I get worried if he will get it again. If my dad ever got cancer again, I'd be crushed."

These words were hard to read. They still are.

I guess there was something about Ford's honesty that touched the hearts of those reading the essays. When a third-grader writes about his father living through cancer and the fear he keeps inside that it may return, people can't help but take notice.

As I considered the essay, I suddenly saw my chances of winning Father of the Year in a whole new light. Shoot, with heartbreaking stuff like that, I was practically a shoo-in! I mean, thanks to Ford, who would have the guts to vote against me?

I started fantasizing about what it might be like to be named Father of the Year. There would surely be some media coverage. Picture in the paper. An interview. I might even be asked to go around to schools and give wise parental advise. "Remember to eat your vegetables," I'd say. "Floss regularly, and give your parents a break. They're doing the best they can!"

Perhaps there would be a bus tour. Or maybe I'd get to wear a crown.

But I was getting ahead of myself. To make it any further in the contest, I had to complete a lengthy questionnaire filled with difficult questions I'd never even considered. The questionnaire wasn't just a page or two; it was more like writing an autobiography. And the probing questions it asked... one would think I was taking out a second mortgage or applying for a job with the FBI. (Was this considered under oath?)

But if I was going to be Father of the Year—and I was damn it!—I had no choice but to fill out the questionnaire and submit it.

While completing the questionnaire, I purposely omitted anything about cancer. That would make it too easy, like taking candy from a baby. I wanted to earn this puppy on my own merits. Sure, Ford's thoughts on cancer had gotten us in the door, but now it was my time to shine!

But who was I kidding? After filling in pages and pages of questions and deciding, often for the very first time, my particular stance on various difficult parenting issues, I figured that was the last I'd hear from the National Center for Fathering. They were surely looking for someone with a better resume.

A couple of weeks passed with no news, and I soon forgot about the whole crown scenario. But then I received a call telling me I'd made it into the final ten! All I had to do was a couple of interviews to see if I would be one of the five finalists.

The final ten? You've got to be kidding.

Perhaps they made a mistake, I thought. Surely that was it. My answers had probably gotten mixed up with one of those dads who coached three of his son's teams a year or was the PTA Treasurer.

On the other hand, who knew how many dads had even filled out the questionnaire? Maybe I'd sneaked in by default. Plus, I'm a writer. If I couldn't do a decent job answering some written questions, I might have to reevaluate my career.

But the next round was an interview. That was another matter altogether. An interview... well, I was bound to screw that up. Like most writers, I tend to be a bit on the introverted side. Oh, I have my moments, but as a general rule, I'm not great at making first impressions.

Of course, if I was able to somehow make it close, by using more voice inflexion and enthusiastic words, well, who knew? After all, I did have that whole "this one may be dead soon" thing going for me.

Two lengthy interviews followed. And, as I had suspected, each ended with some subtle, carefully phrased questions about cancer.

Ka-ching!

Despite my attempts to steer clear of the subject, cancer was still my unfortunate trump card. Thus, I was chosen as one of the five finalists for Oklahoma City's Father of the Year. I'm sure it went something like this: Let's take the guy who taught his daughter to play the bagpipes, the guy who's a stay at home dad for six kids, the guy who volunteers at the children's hospital, the guy who wrote a symphony in honor of each of his kids, and...oh, better throw in the cancer guy.

The five finalists were honored with a very nice banquet at the Oklahoma City Civic Center, hosted by Mr. Canfield and one of those local television anchormen whose name I can never remember. I stood onstage with Ford as the five finalists were announced, and never felt prouder...of my son.

At the end of the day, I was not named Father of the Year, surprise, surprise. The stay at home jerk won. (We like to say there was a problem with "hanging chads.") But I did have some pretty decent broccoli casserole and a great time with Ford.

This was surely one of my fathering highlights, but quite honestly many of my cancer days haven't been nearly as impressive, from a parenting point of view. Parenting is hard enough without cancer. But with cancer, it can be overwhelming.

When I recently asked Ford to describe me, he said I was "sad." I decided to get a second opinion, so I asked Madison if she thought I was sad. And she said, "Duh...you cry like all the time." This was an exaggeration, I think, but the point is well taken.

As my wife recently put it, "Your children deserve to have their father around, to have a normal childhood without all the fear."

And they do. They deserve better.

The problem is, I don't always know how to be better. Most of the time I'm just doing the best I can. Strangely enough, nobody comes knocking on your door to explain how to give your kids a normal childhood when cancer strikes. For the most part, you have to find your own way.

But, for what it's worth, I'm trying harder to be there for them, to step outside my own grief and fear, and to be strong. I'm searching for those moments when their cancer angst slips out, so I can open some dialogue. And I'm trying to let them know there are no guarantees, without making them scared of their own shadows.

I don't always succeed. But perhaps, as I've come to recognize my shortcomings, I'm doing a little better. And maybe, just maybe, the next time around their timelines will simply say, "Dad took us to Six Flags."

LUCKY MAN

Rainbow water glides
peacefully along, a flat plain
holding bird and sun's reflection.

Guitar boy asleep in unstable tent,
not far from worn out buddy,
wrestling asthmatic sputters.

Wife beat a hasty exit, up early
to get that much-needed cup of joe
from some greasy roadside station.

Dog lies still, watching
the morning amble in,
listening to the locusts' program.

Husband out lounging as best he can
in uncomfortable fold-up chair,
considering it all.

Good health comes and goes, yes.
But finding love—that's no given.
So few find contentment there.

Kids grow up fast, test you good,
but there are split-seconds
when all is golden sun right.

What if this moment
could go on and on? But it can't,
you know. It just can't.

The future's possibilities
are helter-skelter scary...
from casket to California.

But today, there's a tent and a lake,
a family and a dog,
reasons to not give up hope.

Jim Chastain   135

15

Gloom, Despair, and Agony

melancholy - *n.* 1. Sadness or depression of the spirits; gloom. 2. Pensive reflection or contemplation. 3. An emotional state characterized by sullenness and outbreaks of violent anger, believed to arise from black bile.
—*American Heritage Dictionary*

Midway on our life's journey, I found myself
   In dark woods, the right road lost. To tell
   About those woods is hard—so tangled and rough
And savage that thinking of it now, I feel
   The old fear stirring: death is hardly more bitter.
   And yet, to treat the good I found there as well
I'll tell you what I saw...
   — from *The Inferno of Dante,* Robert Pinksy, trans.

You know those personality temperament tests you take from time to time? The ones that divide people into four categories: phlegmatic (calm), choleric (angry), sanguine (cheerful), and melancholic (sad)?

Well, I've taken several versions of those tests, and mine always come out the same. Supposedly, I'm melancholic.

I was never particularly happy about this label. (Of course not, you say, you're a melancholic!) For who, when you get right down to it, wants to be known as melancholy? That description implies I am difficult, sulking, and complex, a person who is trouble, insofar as relationships go.

I always believed my personality test results were inaccurate, that there was some inherent flaw in the system. My guess was that there simply weren't enough categories. Sure, I tend to be more melancholy than I do angry, but I'm generally calm and usually quite cheerful, a roll with the punches sort of guy.

But if I were brutally honest, I'd have to admit there have been days, past and present, when my brooding side has emerged—the artistic, emotional, overly critical, self-absorbed, and slightly perfectionist part of me.

As a kid, I was often described as "tender-hearted." I couldn't stand it when bad things happened to someone I knew, or even those I didn't know. I seemed to have a built-in "fairness" meter. (Over time, I learned to compensate for, or hide, this gentle side by building walls of sarcasm and sheer orneriness. My sisters, bless their hearts, bore the brunt of my journey of self-discovery.)

I liked to have time by myself, and I drew a lot when I was alone. I read books that made me feel something, like *Charlotte's Web*, the Roald Dahl collection, and *My Side of the Mountain*. At the movies, I cried easily when things got sad, as if I had been personally wounded. *Old Yeller* just about dealt me a fatal blow, as did *Where the Red Fern Grows*, *Bambi*, and, more recently, *Dances with Wolves*. (After that film, my wife had the pleasure of watching me pull over our car to sob for fifteen minutes. Ask her about it sometime, and she may tell you, if she can stop laughing.)

As a teenager, I developed a wild streak that seemed bent on testing all boundaries of life. No system was sacred; I had to figure it out for myself. Authority was to be questioned. My friends and I had a bold motto: "Anything once."

During that time, I remember going to parties and feeling very alone. I would stand in the middle of a crowd and suddenly have a strong desire to leave. On several occasions, I walked outside and watched those in attendance parading around in their masks, wondering if any of them would miss me. It was then, I suppose, that I began pondering what life was really all about and whether there was any real meaning to it.

I once broke up with a girlfriend on a matter of principle and was so heartbroken when she didn't come crawling back to me, but instead started dating a rich jerk (apparently I wasn't indispensable), that I gave up dating for nearly two years. Relationships were too painful to pursue, and I vowed never to get hurt again.

In later years, I turned to writing and poetry. I have a tendency to turn things over and over in my mind, all the absurdities and wonders of life. I often wondered why things worked out a certain way or how something got so screwed up. Poetry gave me an opportunity to vent.

While the brooding side was not a predominant part of my everyday life, it often appeared. It was part of who I was then and who I am now, a guy who tends to be self-reflective to a fault, with an artistic side and a very dry sense of humor.

During my cancer trials, this side of me, this melancholic nature, suddenly burst forth one day, showing a much darker side than ever before. I plunged into a period of depression that is difficult to understand and much more difficult to talk about openly and honestly.

But what's the point of going through a trial in your life if you don't learn from it and grow in the process? If life's truly "not all about me," perhaps I have a responsibility to share my story with others so they, too, can learn from those experiences.

And so I guess it's time to tell the truth...how I came to chop off my big toe. Not really.

Ready? Okay, here we go...

In the months following my initial cancer diagnosis, I experienced what I now refer to as "brain fog." Now it's hard to explain exactly what brain fog is, but, like a bad haircut, you know it when you've got it.

A brain fog is a self-preserving, protective state your mind lapses into after experiencing a highly traumatic event. I suppose the proper term is post-traumatic shock, but the analogy to fog works best for me.

With brain fog, you're mentally there, most certainly awake, but your brain is sluggish, unable to focus to the same extent it normally would. Something you could easily comprehend on a regular day becomes fuzzy and unclear. You go through the motions of life and decision making without thinking much at all, for any attempt to concentrate is exhausting.

Brain fog is like an out-of-body experience. You're there, and yet you're not. Any Boston Red Sox fan who hears the name Bill Buckner knows exactly what I'm talking about.

My first experience with brain fog occurred after my sister Karyn died in a car wreck at the age of twenty. In the aftermath, I was a walking zombie, more dead than alive. For months, I was often incapable of forming a complete thought without somehow relating it to my sister's death.

I suffered through another bout of brain fog after I was first diagnosed with cancer, and it lasted two or three months. During this time, I had difficulty concentrating on much of anything. The ordeal was so intense it was nearly impossible for me to work or, even worse, to talk with my wife about what we were facing. I was just trying to get through each day.

The fog finally began to lift, as fog tends to do, but then life became extremely busy. I was recovering from surgery and having daily radiation treatments, which completely zapped my strength. Meanwhile, LeAnn and I were both working and trying to keep up with obligations and our kid's activities. Thanksgiving and Christmas were suddenly upon us, along with all the normal busyness and stress of that season. I had a weekly newspaper column to write and was behind at work.

I didn't have a lot of time to think about cancer. We had too much going on.

At this point, I pause to consider the male mid-life crisis, which often takes place between the ages of 35 and 40. Again, it is difficult to describe what a mid-life crisis is, but we know them when we see them, don't we?

A mid-life crisis is usually associated with the perceived death of one's dreams, a lapsing into an existential "so this is it?" state of mind. For a man, this often means opening your eyes one day and finding yourself in a difficult job you never dreamed of doing, in relationships that are dead or at least struggling, or locked in a state of near hopeless indebtedness. Hairlines are disappearing, waistlines are increasing, and deadlines for living the life you've always wanted are long overdue.

Although some of these things did not apply to my situation (the hairline and waistline were a concern), my cancer diagnosis came a few months before turning 38. So I was at the right age for a midlife crisis, if that has anything at all to do with what I experienced.

Anyway, to recap, the holidays had come and gone, and I—a 38 year old, cancerous melancholic, who was squarely within the typical mid-life crisis years—suddenly found myself on the back side of all the busyness. The brain fog was lifting, and I had time to think, to contemplate the "bullet" I had dodged. This, after all, is what a melancholic does.

So what did I think about?

Everything. Every single bit of it. And it was pretty terrifying stuff. My black bile was beginning to build and build.

I thought about my kids. Would I see them grow up, go to the prom, graduate from high school, head off to college, and marry? Madison was nearly eleven. Ford would soon turn eight. How long would they even remember me, if I died?

I thought about LeAnn. We'd had a great marriage, but now we were struggling to even talk to each other. Our intimacy had been replaced by a distant arrangement in which we spent most of our time together trying to make difficult decisions about money and healthcare. Did she find me disgusting, now that I had cancer? She seemed to be dealing with her grief by throwing herself more and more into her work. Was she in for the long haul, or would she pack bags? I'd seen the statistics. Marriage is difficult enough without having your husband get cancer.

I thought about the future and my dreams. I'd wanted to be a writer, someone who wrote books and screenplays and movie reviews and poetry. There was something inside me that was bursting to get out. I wanted to be published and read and understood. I wanted to connect with people in the head and the heart. I wanted to be like Hemingway (minus the bullet in the brain). Had my dreams gone up in smoke?

I thought about work. I had a good job as an attorney for a criminal appeals court, and the pay was decent (for a state government job). I had some good friends and the job gave me an outlet for my creativity, along with a lot of freedom. But I'd gone as far as I would go there, both in rank and in pay. Plus, it was suddenly much more difficult to deal with the stupid things criminals do to innocent people and to themselves. Didn't they know how precious and fleeting life is?

Criminal appeals are probably not the safest place for a melancholic mind to wander about year after year.

To be frank, it was extremely difficult to even go to work. What was the point, I often asked, when I wasn't even sure if I would live another year? Why should I waste what could be my last days sitting in an office? Work was pretty meaningless, when you got right down to it, except for the whole making money part of it.

I thought about my mom and dad. They had already lost one child; how cruel it would be to lose another. A good portion of their joy had been taken away permanently. I wasn't sure they'd make it through if it happened again.

I thought about my friendships, how much pain they brought. The closer I was to someone, the more it seemed to hurt. I had become a sort of cancer myself, spreading tears and sadness to everyone to whom I was significantly connected and loved. One has to have friends in life to get by, but sometimes I longed to be a hermit.

I thought about money, how my condition was putting a financial burden on my family. I was like Jimmy Stewart in *It's a Wonderful Life,* worth more dead than alive.

I thought about my next checkup in Houston, just a month or so away. What if the cancer returned? I was still in danger. And there were other things going on, too. Issues with people, and church, and time commitments.

These were a few of my thoughts and concerns, some of the predominant ones.

As I considered my life, I began slipping into an emotional funk. I was surely fighting it, reminding myself of how lucky I was, how much I had, how the cancer was probably gone, stuff like that. But the bottom line is my life felt very tenuous and small, and I had no more room for turmoil.

And then there was the "triggering event," that one additional thing that sent me over the edge, the straw that broke the camel's back. What happened? Well, that's another story. Let's just leave it at this: One more level of stress was added to my already fragile emotional condition and as a result my generally positive foundation crumbled.

I, Humpty Dumpty, had a great fall.

Depression set in, big time. I was lost in a valley of despair like none I had ever known. The weight of the world seemed to be resting on my chest. I could hardly eat, sleep, or recognize myself in the mirror. I was a complete stranger.

I experienced what they used to sing about on *Hee-Haw* (undoubtedly one of the worst television shows in history)—"Gloom, despair, and agony on me. Deep dark depression, excessive misery"—in other words, brain fog times five.

It is important to recognize that cancer, or any similarly calamitous event, can use up so much of one's emotional energy that there's no room for anything else to go wrong. Stress takes its toll, and too much stress at any particular time can cause a major crash. No matter what anyone may tell you, life is not *really* a bowl of cherries. Bad things happen to good people everyday. And cancer, like heart disease, a bad automobile accident, or Alzheimer's, will test your stress meter, to see how much you can take.

So what do you do when you find you've sunk into an alarming state of depression? Well, I'm no psychologist, and I make no promise of a sure fire cure. But here's what I did.

First, I began reading about depression, what it is, how long it lasts, what to do about it. There are hundreds of books and internet articles on the subject, and you'll have no problem finding one to fit your particular circumstances.

Second, I talked about it. I began by reestablishing communication channels with my wife. LeAnn and I have always been blessed with the ability to have deep, meaningful conversation. Cancer had changed that somewhat, but now I opened up like I never had before in our marriage, telling her some dark details of my journey and my current reality. This was difficult, and I made some mistakes. But as a result, we entered a deeper level of intimacy than we'd ever experienced.

I also talked with friends. I am blessed with a good group of friends around me, including several whom I meet with regularly. I shared my struggles with them, as best I could. They listened to me, let me bleed and, for the most part, did not feel a pressing need to offer any save-the-day advice. The chance to let some of my pain out to friends, little by little, helped.

I also began meeting with a counselor so I could talk openly about my wounds and the masks I sometimes hide behind. It felt good to tell it all to a disinterested party, without having to worry about repercussions. The counselor encouraged me and challenged me to be more open and honest about my struggles.

Third, I wrote about it. I journaled my emotional battle. I wrote poems, some very positive, but some bitter and caustic. I began sending e-mails to friends and family to keep them updated on my situation. At some point, I began planning this book. Writing has always been therapeutic for me.

Fourth, I continued searching for God. I prayed often about my struggles and asked for strength. I began journaling on the Psalms and found myself connecting with the authors and their various predicaments and points of view. Our stories intersected quite often, and there I found moments of peace, camaraderie, and hope.

Fifth, I reached out. During my depression, there was something mysteriously healing about the sense of touch. I would hug my kids until they were about to gag with embarrassment. To touch my wife's hand or shoulder or pinkie toe for that matter was a slice of pure heaven. I made a point to hug my extended family, to shake hands whenever possible, to pat a friend on the back.

And finally, I waited. Depression is often short-lived, typically lasting only two or three months. Knowing this, I clung to my family and struggled through each day.

At some point in time, thanks in large part to the support I received from loved ones—especially my ever-patient wife—I made it through the darkness. And as I did, I realized, once again, that I had learned much about myself and the gift of life.

I learned that I take too much for granted. I'd been living life as if I would be here forever, or at least a good eighty years. But this is not a given, as my sister Karyn and two of my prior bosses have demonstrated. Today is a gift, and I'd better make the most of it. Today, there is hope.

I learned I was not immune to depression. Many people with strong faith have reportedly experienced depression. C.S. Lewis. Bill Hybels. Brendon Manning. Parker Palmer. Henry Nouwen. The list goes on and on. Jesus himself was tormented by grief and anguish in the Garden of Gethsemane. My religious beliefs didn't exempt me or anyone else from struggles with depression.

I learned to be more open and honest, with myself and with those closest to me. It is a frightening thing to let it all hang out, to let your darkness come into the light. People can hurt you when you tell it like it is, but such risk-taking can also bring great rewards when the gamble of authenticity pays off. For the most part, we all want to know and be known. And so, the question isn't whether I should tell someone who I really am. The question is who are the people in whom I can safely confide.

I learned my emotional needs are as important as my spiritual or physical needs. If I am losing my temper too much, worrying all the time, or feeling the blues, I have the responsibility to recognize that fact and address it. I need to build daily stress reducers into my life, like spending time with friends, date nights, journaling, exercise, etc.

I learned it's not shameful to seek professional counseling.

My period of depression wasn't about crying, "Look at poor me." No, it was more like saying, "Look at how wonderful life is. Too bad it can't last."

But at some point, you realize your days on earth are numbered, and it's not worth it to let another one go by just because it's all going to end some day. Live the days you've been given, and enjoy them as much as you can. Write poetry, call your friends, be romantic, throw a party, have deep conversations, worship, encourage someone, read a good book, go see a movie, chat over coffee, and love.

In the end, depression can be a positive thing. A friend's counselor once told her, "Thank God for cancer," for it had brought her and her mother much closer together. This has been my experience, too, in my battle with depression.

So I raise my glass now and propose a toast. "Thank God for cancer and for this period of depression. No matter what happens from here, I am a better person because of the many lessons I learned along the way."

And, finally, let me just say it right now. To my sisters, Lori, Cindy, and Karyn—I'm sorry I was such a bothersome pest.

ALREADY GONE

Who's to say the golden sun
isn't forever hidden by ominous clouds?
That the grass isn't permanently withered brown
and scattered about by the chapped-lip wind?
That swimming pool's once cool blue
hasn't been replaced by murky gray?

> The happiness that was.
> The lives unhindered by diagnosis.

Who's to say any semblance
of summer warmth will return?
That the sandy beaches of yesterday
will ever host another suntanned visitor?
That the baseball mitt will come down
from the dusty attic?

> The end of silver-linings.
> We who never knew a breaking point.

The dog no longer prances
in back yard's freshly mowed lines.
The cat chooses musty garage
over cozy apple tree shade.
And hope, once shattered,
gives way to stale survival.

16

You Say It's Your Birthday

A friend of mine was about to turn forty and really dreading it. I was sitting across from her one day as she began mourning the loss of her youth. She was "feeling down" about the passage into another decade of life. It was "only yesterday" when she left college.

"Where did my thirties go?" she asked. "Forty seems so...old."

Blah, blah, blah, I thought.

Now don't get me wrong. I like this person. She had been there for me during my health crisis. Plus, I completely understood where she was coming from—people my age tend to obsess about getting older all the time. It's what we do.

But still, her existentialism seemed a bit insensitive to me, a guy who had been struggling with cancer. At the time, I was just hoping to make it through another year. *She should be thankful for having the opportunity to turn forty!* I fumed to myself. *It's better than the alternative.*

And so, as she sighed and whined and grimaced and felt sorry for herself, I began having fantasies about stuffing a nasty oversized gym sock into her mouth, one with sweat and fuzzballs and dog drool all over it.

That, I mused, *would give her some perspective.*

Emotions can get out of whack when you have cancer. No matter how even-tempered you may be, spend a few years with the disease and you'll probably struggle with the desire to smack a best friend or choke a close relative.

That's how it was with me anyway. After struggling with cancer for three years, I was an emotional wreck. Instead of empathizing with my friend who was feeling down about her age, all I could do was get angry. Cancer had gone so far as to rob me of my God-given right as an American to gripe about getting older!

And yet, I was sad and gloomy on my fortieth birthday too, but for other reasons. For I spent my fortieth birthday lying flat on my back in a Houston hospital bed, trying to recover from a nine-hour surgery on my right arm, my fourth cancer surgery in two and a half years.

Insofar as sad and gloomy occasions go, this one took the birthday cake.

The cancer had returned for its third attempt on my life. A long and painful surgery had ended late in the afternoon on the day before my birthday. After spending hours in recovery, I was wheeled into my hospital room about 9 p.m., just three hours before I was to turn over a new decade.

My first conscious birthday memory was at 2 a.m., when a nurse woke me to take vital signs.

You know how it works in hospitals, don't you? Hospitals are the last place in the world you'd ever go for a good night's sleep. At hospitals, sleep is viewed as the silent killer. Every two hours or so, some extremely noisy person enters your room to make sure you're still breathing. (This helps to pad the hospital's survival rate.)

Anyway, as the middle-of-the-night nurse took my pulse, blood pressure, and temperature, it suddenly dawned on me that it was my birthday. I even mumbled something to that effect, which, in retrospect, turned out to be a very bad idea.

After the nurse left, I couldn't go back to sleep. I was piping hot and sweating like an aerobics instructor, despite the fact that the room was absolutely frigid and a fan was blowing cold air directly on me. (This is one of those freaky anesthesia things you can never quite understand.)

I turned on the TV. My choices were pretty bad. But then I turned to

PBS, which was airing the latest Broadway production of *Oklahoma!*, starring Hugh Jackman. This may sound horrible to you, but for an Oklahoman like me, one who has seen that particular musical performed live at least twenty times, it was like stumbling upon the Holy Grail. For some reason, it made me feel closer to home. So I settled in to watch, although I kept passing out every now and then from the residual anesthesia.

LeAnn was sleeping nearby in a foldout bed. The TV wasn't bothering her, but she'd been having fits with the room temperature, which was probably hovering around 58 degrees. (The next night, she would give me an ultimatum: I could either relinquish control of the thermostat or spend the night alone.)

About 4 a.m., as *Oklahoma!* was winding down, four nurses entered my room. Apparently, this was the nightshift quartet. One of the nurses had been told it was my birthday, so she'd brought in the choir to spread a little joy before they went off duty.

The nurses started singing "Happy Birthday" at a volume that was, quite frankly, terrifying. The leader of the quartet, who was likely a part time opera singer, was really getting into it.

This was a nice gesture, I suppose. But at four o'clock in the morning—with me half-sick and my wife trying to get some brief moments of sleep between vital checks and shivers—it was sheer madness.

I tried to shush them, to keep them from waking LeAnn. It was nearly Christmas, after all, and she was liable to deck their halls. But I only succeeded in getting them to turn down the volume a few decibels.

After they were gone, LeAnn said with that tone she uses, "Tell me that wasn't your nurses singing 'Happy Birthday.'"

"That wasn't my nurses singing 'Happy Birthday,'" I lied.

"Good, because I was about to hurt someone," she said.

They had barely escaped with their lives.

At six a.m., the shift changed, and a male nurse named Raven entered my room. I already knew Raven from my surgery the previous year, and he is great, especially for a male nurse named Raven.

"I hear it's your birthday," Raven said, in his quiet, scratchy way.

"Yup."

"Mine, too," he said. "Well, tomorrow."

"Really?"

"Uh-huh. I'm turning forty," he said.

"You're kidding! *I'm* forty today!"

"Really? Man, this is no place for your fortieth. You're supposed to be havin' a party."

"We're celebrating next week."

"Well, my party's on Friday, and I can't wait!" Raven said.

"This is *so* weird, Raven. We could be twins separated at birth."

This was funnier if you'd been there. Raven is a short African American with dreadlocks and a high pitched Michael Jackson voice. I couldn't be a whiter shade of pale, and I have short hair and a fairly deep voice.

"'63 was a good year," I said.

"'63? I was born in '64!" he replied.

At that point, I paused. Perhaps it was the anesthesia, but I just couldn't figure out a way that Raven, who was born exactly one year and one day after me, could possibly be turning forty on the day after I was. I'm no mathematician, but the numbers didn't add up.

I thought of every possibility. Leap year. Being held back in school. Incubators. A coma. Cryogenics. I even recalculated my own birthday, making sure my parents hadn't screwed it up. But still...nothing.

I had no choice but to help Raven face the cold hard truth.

"Dude, you're turning 39," I said.

"No, I'm not! I'm turning forty!" he answered, firmly.

"I don't think so," I laughed.

"Listen, my brother's, like, two years older than me, and he was forty-one on his last birthday..."

I gave him an amused look.

"Hey, I wouldn't be having my 40th birthday party if I wasn't sure," he said, in a panicked way.

"Well, you might want to go add it up or call your Mom or something," I suggested.

So Raven left, looking like he'd been punched in the gut. I didn't hear from him for several hours, which was odd. He was usually in my room every hour or so. I figured he was waiting on a fax from his birth hospital.

When he finally reentered my room, he seemed a little down. I didn't say anything though. I'd already rained on his parade enough for one day.

He approached with his head hanging low. "You were right," he said, dejectedly. "I'm turning 39."

"Yeah..." I said, pausing to show the depth of my pain. "Sorry, man."

And I was.

"It's okay," he said.

And then he smiled. Perhaps as he saw me lying there, he realized there were worse things in the world than being 39 rather than 40.

What a joy it is to be everyone's barometer for what can go wrong in life!

My strange birthday continued with a visit from my doctor. She explained how my surgery had gone. The cancer was confined to my triceps muscle, but this time there had been three tumors instead of one. One by my elbow. One in the middle of the triceps. And one more, the "ominous" tumor, closer to my armpit.

Needless to say, this wasn't great news. The cancer had moved beyond its point of origin, uncomfortably close to my lungs. But she thought they'd gotten it all.

I was quiet. The stakes kept climbing higher and higher. If the cancer returned again, they would take my arm.

Noticing my somber state and knowing it was my birthday, my doctor asked, "Do you like sushi?"

I'd never eaten sushi. I'm from Oklahoma, after all, and ordering sushi there had never seemed like the safest bet.

"I don't know. I've never tried it."

"Would you like me to pick you up some?" she asked. "We're going to this place that has great sushi."

Hmmm...Would I like to eat raw fish less than eighteen hours after major surgery, when the only thing I had put into my stomach so far was 7-Up? Would I like to try some new exotic food I had never dared to eat under normal conditions, a food that had never sounded the least bit desirable?

"Sure," I said. It wasn't going to make me feel any worse than I already did. Plus, if anything went wrong, I was already at the hospital.

One hour later, I was sitting in my hospital bed eating sushi for the first time in my life. It was...good, although probably not something I would purposely choose. But at least I could cross that one off my list of things to do before I die. Next it was that elusive Academy Award.

Late in the afternoon, a physical therapist arrived to take me for a birthday walk around my hospital floor. This was like suddenly being told it was time to climb Mount Everest or win the Tour de France. At that point, it was a daunting task to even think about sitting up in bed.

My surgery had been extensive. The triceps muscle from my right arm had been removed, approximately one third of my upper arm. The muscle had been replaced by one from my back, along with a football shaped strip of skin from my back. My arm and back were aching from the incisions and stitches.

I'd also had a skin graft taken from my right leg, and my left hip had a mysterious swelling. I had three drains hanging from me—two in my back and one in my arm. I had a catheter in, which was a bit confining, and an IV in my left arm, attached to various bags of medicine hanging from one of those coat racks on wheels. Plus, my stomach was queasy, for obvious sushi-related reasons.

So what do you do when you have three bags, an IV, and a catheter hanging from you, along with a missing area of skin on your leg, swelling on your hip, a queasy stomach, and stitches all up and down your arm and leg? Why, you go for a stroll!

The physical therapist was a nice-looking woman, approximately my age. She and a nurse proceeded to strip me naked, which was bizarre and humiliating, but necessary to prepare for my walk. So there I stood in my birthday suit, looking like a frail version of Frankenstein's monster, while they replaced my old hospital gown with two fresh ones. They fastened the two gowns at my side in a way that resembled a silly dress. As a result, I could go for a walk and hold my head high!

I made it twice around my floor, which was a miracle considering how horrible I felt. It was exhausting work. When I was finished, I plopped down in a chair for the rest of the evening, making sure to keep my knees together at all times, as is proper when you're wearing a dress.

As my 40th birthday drew to a close, I sat in the same chair contemplating the events of the last few days (including a theft from our hotel room on the night before surgery that resulted in the loss of all of LeAnn's jewelry). LeAnn was in the bathroom taking a shower, and I was feeling blue.

Where was all this going? Four surgeries in two and a half years—what would the next two and a half hold? I wanted to remain optimistic, but it was becoming increasingly difficult. Things weren't going my way.

How would I handle myself when we returned home? Would I be depressed? What would I do about work? And where was God in all of this?

Sara, my nurse, walked in. Sara had been with me during all three of my Houston surgeries and had been a positive influence from the very beginning. She'd been helpful and informative during my first stay, and we'd had an encouraging talk during my second stay. This time around, she'd been a little less chatty, but I didn't think too much about it. She was probably busy. Besides, I was in no mood to talk either.

Sara began changing my sheets, while I remained in the chair, deep in thought. Apparently sensing my mood, Sara approached and looked me straight in the eyes as she asked, "What are you doing?"

"I don't know...just thinking."

"About what?"

"Oh, you know...everything."

Sara took my hand. "When I saw you sitting here feeling sorry for yourself, I knew I had to talk to you." She paused. "Listen, I've never told anyone this before..."

Sara then told me the heartbreaking story of how her husband had died the year before, just a few weeks after I had been released from the hospital the last time. His death was totally unexpected. He had passed away in his sleep one night without warning as he lay in bed, the victim, if I remember right, of an aneurysm. Sara had been left grieving with two sons still in high school and a full time job to hold down.

Tears were rolling from her eyes as she spoke, but she still managed to smile.

"Oh my God, Sara. How did you do it? How did you get by?" I asked.

"It was hard. Very, very hard," she admitted. "I took six weeks off from work, to get everything in order. But it was horrible, and I was sad. I woke up every morning and just cried and cried. You know, I'd been working with cancer patients for years, but this was the first time I really understood what they go through."

I nodded. We'd both reached that level of misery that enabled us to communicate on a different level. Sara "got it." She understood my deep pain and grief and loneliness. And I understood hers.

Sara continued, "But I couldn't give up. I had to work! I have two boys to raise. They'd lost their father. They were hurting and needed me to be strong for them. I didn't have a choice. I had to go on."

My kids needed me to be strong, too.

"Life is hard," Sara continued. "It doesn't always go your way. But you've got to keep going. You can't give up. I get up every morning and fast and pray for two hours. This helps me. You can do it too. Don't lose your faith."

"Do you still cry?" I asked.

"Yes...every morning. I'm very lonely. But God has a plan, I think. It may be difficult, but I'm doing my best to see it through."

It was a powerful moment, one I will never be able to fully explain. I was feeling about as low as I ever had, unable to see beyond my circumstances. And I'd been specifically thinking about where I would go from there, and whether or not God would be there with me.

Timing is everything, they say. For me, the timing of this moment—with a person I barely knew about a topic she had never before shared—was significant. My birthday present that day was an unexpected and much-needed pep-talk.

God has never spoken to me audibly. In fact, most of the time, when I have yearned for one of those "God spoke to me" moments we sometimes hear about, God has instead remained eerily silent. But there have also been those times when God seems to communicate through timely events or the encouraging words of friends.

Through my heartbreaking conversation with Sara, I sensed God's presence, saying, "Yes, I'm here. Yes, there's a plan. Be strong. Give it your best and see this through."

Of course, skeptics would call it sheer coincidence that I was thinking of God and then interpreted what happened to me in that light. And perhaps they'd be right. Plus, I can't completely rule out the possibility that it had something to do with that birthday sushi.

FROM THE WINDOW

the world looks almost peaceful
from this watchtower room where i'm quarantined
outside there's a constant drip drip drip of rain
as from a distant eye behind the somber clouds
forty yards away raisin men work in drizzle and fog
constructing a new building for new people like me
i imagine a little boy with sad eyes there now
we're waving to each other

to the west the haunted hotels
filled with outpatients and aching families
form a sorry skyline above the medical plaza
the smell of paprika and curry overpowers
but not here where hospital food will soon arrive
inching forward i see downtown houston not far
from what was once enron field where
my son and I may someday watch a ballgame

alone here with my thoughts and memories
and these alarming tubes sticking out of me
i'm like the high school kid no one remembers
friends and family phone from long distances
but there are no familiar faces nearby
no one to touch or hold or send a smile my way
so for now i sit looking out from the window
while time's clutch remains stuck in neutral

17

Moving On

My family attended a Southern Baptist church for many years. Not one of those ultra-conservative types, but a somewhat moderate church that actually saw women as persons who are gifted and valued by God. (That is, unless they're lesbians.)

But we had recently made the painful, yet freeing, move to a non-denominational church. This new church seemed to be a better fit for us *at that time*, which is to say that it was filled with people who were, as a general rule, as screwed up as we were.

One of the things that first attracted us to this new church, beyond its non-Baptist ways, was that we were *completely* undercover there. At my former church, we were well-known fixtures, having served in various "high profile" positions, whatever that means. But at this new church, we were nobodies. I was just another new guy. Only a handful of people knew me by name, and fewer still knew I'd been battling cancer.

That felt incredibly refreshing. For a couple of hours each week, I was no longer the "cancer guy." I was just Jim or the "recovering Baptist" or "so what was your name again?"

Normally, I wouldn't want to be so anonymous. For the most part, we all want to be known. But these weren't normal times. These were the cancer years. Being a complete stranger felt rather good. Plus, it was church. The more you're known at a church, the more likely it is you'll be asked to sign up for something.

But as time passed and we met more people at the new church, the word slowly began to trickle out about me and my darned health issues. Try as I might to plug up the breach, I couldn't keep the dam of information from bursting.

I'm not sure how it happened. I suppose somebody knew somebody else whose aunt had a neighbor who was concerned about my cancer. But before long, the rumor mill started and someone on staff heard about my...situation.

My precious anonymity was gone, just like that.

The first time I realized "they knew" was during a phone call. The pastor's wife called to ask LeAnn and I to talk in church about the struggles we'd recently experienced. The topic that day was to be "Seasons of Marriage," and we were to fill the "in sickness and in health" slot.

Incidentally, as a general rule this is not a slot you want to be asked to fill.

I didn't receive the phone call. LeAnn did. I was in the bathroom getting dressed, brushing my teeth, or...reading. But I could hear what was going on out there. LeAnn was saying how we would love to speak on the topic, that we hoped our struggle would be meaningful to others, etc.

Meanwhile, I was having a different reaction. My mind was racing, my stomach was churning, my heart was beginning to sink. My cancer was no longer a secret. I'd been outed!

I had liked being unknown there. I had liked it very much.

Why is this bothering me? I asked myself.

Perhaps it was denial. But no, that couldn't be. I was sufficiently "dealing" with the cancer. I wasn't ignoring it, like it had never happened. In fact, I talked about it all the time. No, it was something else.

Perhaps these were my last remnants of grief. Yeah, I'd been hiding from people to a certain extent, looking for a safe haven, someplace where I wouldn't receive the "oh-my-gosh you're the guy with cancer" look. This new church had been a temporary oasis from the total paradigm shift I'd experienced since my cancer diagnosis. I could play the part of the old Jim there, the total macho stud I used to be. (Really...ask anyone.) There, I wasn't the poster child for what could go wrong in life.

But suddenly all that had changed.

When I shared this with LeAnn, she suggested we call the pastor's wife and tell her we just weren't ready to talk about our experiences yet.

That wasn't the point. I'd always known my dirty little secret would get out someday. I'd just wanted to enjoy the ride while I could. Now that the cat was out of the bag, it was time to move on, time to face the music and try to apply the lessons I'd learned along my cancer journey. And that meant getting out in the world again, living my life, and sharing my experiences with others.

The only other choice was to withdraw. To hide. To disengage. To deliberately choose to stagnate, which was the opposite of moving on.

So we decided to speak that weekend. And it was a good experience. Oh sure, there were a few tough moments—I had a hard time getting through portions of the talk, especially those dealing with my family— but with LeAnn's help the job got done. I shared brief glimpses of some of the things I've shared in this book, although I'm pretty sure I never mentioned the *ménage à trois* or penis farting incidents.

In the last service, when we were finished, several rows actually gave us a standing ovation, the only one I've ever received in my life. Here, it seems, was my Tour de France victory lap. But instead of riding a bike, I was standing in front of a bunch of people I didn't really know, pouring out my wounded heart.

Judging by the comments we received afterward, our story connected with several people. But why? It's not like I'm a seasoned public speaker, and I certainly don't have cancer all figured out. Why did strangers cry along with me? And why did I feel such relief after briefly sharing about our journey?

What, exactly, happened that weekend?

It must have something to do with a deeply-felt human need to know and be known. We all want our lives to count for something; we all want to matter. After all, no man is an island. We need to experience a personal connection with others, no matter how much you tell yourself otherwise.

There's a reason why times of extended isolation can cause a person to lose his or her mind. As has been observed, it's not good for man or woman to be alone.

But here's the paradox: at times cancer seems to run counter to that idea. Although we need people to be there for us when cancer strikes, the horror of the disease often makes us want to go into isolation—to keep to ourselves and hide away all the dirty details of our messed-up lives, all the embarrassing and sad stuff that's so difficult to share. It's a coping mechanism, I think, to avoid all the strange reactions and stress that "talking about it" creates.

The problem, however, is that's not living. If we can't speak to others about who we are and what we've learned along the way, we might as well start planning our funerals.

Cancer robs a person of so much. It steals health, dreams, joy, future, bank accounts, time, the ability to think clearly, and quite often relationships. It leaves one with anger, fear, sorrow, and an overriding sense of exhaustion, worthlessness, and futility. And if we're not careful, it may take away our hope.

In order to counteract all this negativity, we *must*, at some point, move on. That may sound simplistic, but it's true. We've got to reclaim our lives, no matter what may or may not happen in the future; no matter the diagnosis. We must accept this unfortunate turn of events for what it is, and go forward with everything we've got.

We need to come up with a plan and see it through.

In the book *The Anatomy of Hope*, Dr. Jerome Groopman discusses how critical planning is to the process of retaining hope. He writes, "Instilling hope in the brain involves setting a firm goal and anticipating the reward of living with the dream fulfilled." And part of that goal-setting means taking control of our circumstances, so we aren't, as Dr. Groopman puts it, "entirely at the mercy of forces outside (ourselves)."

This is called moving on.

So your health is bad…What are you going to do about it?

So your dreams have gone up in smoke…Dream new ones.

So you're often panicked and joyless…Choose to do something you love to do and spend time with those you love.

There comes a time when we must graduate from Cancer Screwed Up My Life 101.

But it's a choice, you know…moving on. Reclaiming our lives and engaging others once again. It doesn't just happen like magic. We must plan deliberately.

Case in point. I was at work one day, having just returned from a particularly brutal cancer stay in Houston, when a friend told me one of our coworkers had been laid off. The State of Oklahoma, like many other states, had been experiencing massive budget shortfalls. Layoffs were inevitable—the money simply wasn't there.

Someone had to be let go. And Anna was one of the unfortunate ones dealt a devastating blow.

Anna had been at our office longer than anyone else. In fact, she'd been working there since before I graduated from law school.

Anna had an incredible work ethic. She was the first person to arrive at the office in the morning, and the last to go home. She hardly ever missed a day. She rarely took vacation time and was almost never sick. Anna was a hard worker who kept her nose to the grindstone. She didn't fraternize much, but stayed focused on the task at hand.

Because I didn't work directly with her, I can't say how productive Anna was. But she seemed quite competent, and I never heard anyone complain.

But Anna was a loner. As far as I knew, she'd never been married. She had strong religious beliefs that kept her busy and active at church, but at the office she seldom joined in when our morale boosting events were scheduled. Indeed, she seemed to frown upon them.

Anna was an enigma. So I wasn't completely surprised that she was the unfortunate one to get laid off when a cut had to be made. Whether or not it was deliberate, Anna had failed to connect with those around her. So when push came to shove, she had no close friends to go to bat for her.

Later, I was in my office working when I saw Anna walking down the hallway, heading my way. It was her next-to-last day at work, and she was going from office to office, delivering mail.

It was lunchtime, and most of the people at work were gone. Anna had probably chosen that time on purpose to avoid human contact. (I would have done the same thing.) But I had remained at work.

What an awkward situation!

As Anna made her way to my office, I had to make an uncomfortable, split-second decision. The way I saw it, I had two choices: 1) I could accept my mail from Anna and exchange safe, surface-level pleasantries, or 2) I could take a risk and talk to Anna directly about her situation.

But why choose the riskier road? Sure this was a bad break for Anna, but I had problems of my own. I'd just missed a month of work because of cancer. Case files were piled on my desk, and I didn't feel like working on any of them. I was an emotional wreck, struggling to make it through each day.

But so was she.

To engage or not engage. That was the question.

The problem was I had never had a lengthy discussion of any type with Anna over the years. We'd worked in different areas on different things. We had smiled and said hi when passing, but that was it. Although her intensity seemed a bit postal at times, in reality I didn't know her at all.

It would be a difficult conversation, and I didn't always handle those well. But cancer had reminded me that the difficult conversations are often the most important of all. People who have had bad things happen to them need to know they matter.

The human thing to do was to be real. To talk to Anna. To treat her with the dignity she deserved.

Anna entered my office smiling. She handed me my mail and asked her standard question, "How's the family?"

I told her they were fine, even though she didn't know them. As she turned to go, I said, "Anna, I heard what happened, and I'm so sorry. I mean, you've worked here forever and then this happens out of the blue..."

She turned and looked me squarely in the eyes, deep into my soul. With a quivering voice, she let down the walls she'd built. "Yes, it was quite a shock," she said. "I'm not even sure it's sunk in yet. I was getting ready for vacation, a mission trip with my church, and then this...

I nodded, not offering any save-the day advice. I just listened.

"I've tried to keep my mind focused on the trip, but...This is quite a wake-up call."

"So, what are you going to do?" I asked.

Anna sat down and spoke from her heart. We had a twenty-minute conversation, approximately twenty times longer than any we'd ever had. During that time, I discovered that many of my perceptions about Anna were wrong.

Sure, Anna was quiet and serious. But she was also kind and giving. She had deep religious beliefs, but she was no fanatic. Indeed, her faith was strong. She firmly believed she would land on her feet. "I have good days in my future," she said. She explained how she'd been given the opportunity to find what was important. But for now, she would go on her mission trip and serve others.

Anna then asked about my cancer. So I shared some of the details of my latest surgery, along with some of my hopes and fears.

Anna and I had a great conversation, one that never would have happened if I hadn't chosen to engage. My cancer experiences had allowed me to empathize with her in a way I might not have otherwise. I felt better about myself after our conversation than I had in some time. I hope Anna felt better, too.

Later, I wondered why I don't do this sort of thing more often. Two virtual strangers had connected that afternoon, simply by taking a risk. We'd experienced "community," that illusive state where people allow each other to matter.

What a gift we can give to others by simply listening to their stories. By stepping into their shoes. And what a gift we give to ourselves in the meantime.

A week later, I learned that Anna had donated all of her sick leave to me. As I said before, Anna hardly ever missed work and had been working at the Court forever. Consequently, she had hundreds of hours of sick leave built up. Because I was nearly out of sick leave, thanks to my continuous trips to Houston for cancer treatments, Anna's gift was a true blessing.

My little risk was already paying back a hundred times over.

But the story doesn't end there. About a month after Anna had left work, I received a call from a friend, who also worked for the State, but in a different branch.

"I've got a woman coming in for an interview today," he said, "and I think you might know her. She used to work for you guys. Her name is Anne."

"Anne?" I said. "I don't know any..."

He interrupted. "No, wait. It's Anna."

My heart jumped.

"Uh-yes. I know her," I said.

"Well, tell me about her. We've got a job opening, and she's applied. She's got a good shot at it, unless you have something to tell me..."

I was suddenly the person who could make or break Anna's immediate future.

I went on to say every possible thing I could think of in Anna's favor. I was upfront, telling my friend that Anna was quiet and tends to keep to herself. But she was also a hard worker, who never missed work, etc.

The long and the short of it is this—my friend hired Anna. Not for that job (someone from the inside made a lateral move), but for another job that opened that same week at a higher salary than the job for which she interviewed.

Choosing to engage makes all the difference. What happened between Anna and me that day was not all that different from what happened when LeAnn and I spoke at church about our cancer journey. We shared the intimate details of our story with one another. The listeners became part of that story by hearing it and then responding with their own stories.

I guess that is what *true* community means. We can talk and talk to someone about what we know, what we've done, and where we've been, and he or she will look at us with a vacant stare. "Good for you, buddy," they will say, while yawning and thinking of practically anything else.

But when we tell our stories—the real stuff that happens to us with all the attendant pains, joy, and emotions—they begin to identify, to connect. "I've been there, too," they think. "I know what that feels like."

But such communication is a two-way street. Sometimes, by simply listening, a person actually receives more than he or she gives.

In a book I recently read, the author discusses how knowing and being known goes to the very core of life. His theory is we can only be loved to the extent that we are known.

With cancer, I had been comfortable living in the shadows. Being obscure. Not being known. And all lessons aside, I still want to rid myself of the whole cancer freak show at times. But I can't. It's part of who I am. The question is what to do with it.

For me, moving on started with a risky conversation with Anna, a conversation that became one of my most rewarding experiences in years.

It started with the decision to tell my story to others in church, a decision that led to a standing ovation and real conversations with new people

I never would have had otherwise.

It started with a small lump in my arm, and it ends who knows where?

I survived cancer, at least so far, but I never won the Tour de France. Few have.

All I know is it's time to reclaim my life. It's time to engage others. It's time to move on.

THE LAST VOLLEYBALL GAME

There is a last volleyball game
When the sun sinks on the horizon
And the gang all heads off for a Corona

Oh that the game could last
That stamina would not falter
That approaching darkness might be overcome

We've heard of such stories
A chariot rushes down from silvery clouds
And whisks away our protagonist

Could it ever be so
We all want to believe
That dreams really do come true

Once there was a boy
And a ball and a net and a team
He served and did not know the outcome

But the final point eventually comes
The ball goes up in the air
And lands on one side or the other

Win or lose the game suddenly ends
One hasn't a choice in such things
Walking away you miss it already

18

Afterword

More than two years have passed since I finished writing this book. A lot has happened during that time—so much in fact that this book just wouldn't be complete without bringing you up to speed on the latest changes in my health. Hold on, though, for it's not very pretty.

When we last said goodbye, it was the beginning of 2004, and I was trying to recuperate from a rather nasty surgery that had left my arm permanently disabled and at about 50% of its normal strength. I now call that period the good old days. For even though there were challenges, life, for the most part, was fairly normal.

We'd added a Golden Retriever, Gracie, to the family. (We love her dearly now, but back then, during her puppy days, she nearly finished us off.) And LeAnn and I were even able to sneak away for a trip to a beautiful resort in Playa Del Carmen, Mexico in early June. I commemorated that trip earlier with my poem, *The Last Volleyball Game*.

The poem is a tribute to a funny story that happened during our Mexico vacation. Some guys at our resort would meet each afternoon for a beach volleyball game. I wanted so badly to join them, but was hesitant, due to my bum arm. But LeAnn, knowing how much I loved to play the game, encouraged me to go out and "improvise."

The problem, of course, was that I had no triceps in my right arm. This meant, quite literally, that I could not raise my arm straight above my head. It takes triceps to do that, you see, and if I tried my arm would simply fall like a rock to my side.

This poses a problem for volleyball because of all the setting up one has to do. But I improvised, finding all kinds of ways to make it work. I would hit the ball one-handed, or dig it underhanded, using both hands. Given my circumstances, I was doing some miraculous work out there, as God is my witness.

But then it came my turn to serve. I couldn't serve over-handed, like I'd used to, so I attempted the underhand method, straight into a strong wind.

Now the first part of the underhand serve relies almost entirely on the biceps. And that was good, for my biceps were intact and as strong as ever.

What I hadn't taken into account was the follow through, when your arm impacts the ball and then travels forward and upward in a straight motion. This is triceps territory. And so, when I struck the ball and then followed through, I had no muscle to stop my arm from continuing forward. My arm never stopped until my hand smacked me squarely in the face, nearly knocking me down.

Dazed and with my sunglasses hanging crooked off my nose, I collected myself, embarrassed to see how many people had witnessed what had to have been the funniest serve in the history of modern volleyball. But to my amazement, nobody had seen it.

Unfortunately, we won the point, and it was my turn to serve again. Uh-oh...Knowing where this was going, I concocted a quick lie, telling my teammates I was tired and needed a replacement. They looked at me incredulously. We were the reigning court champs, mind you. *Nobody* left when their team held this position.

We decided to take a quick water break. So I walked over to LeAnn, who was also wondering why I'd suddenly stopped playing. "The wind's too strong on this side," I said. "I wound up hitting myself in the face during my serve."

"Can't you do it another way?" she asked.

I thought about it for a minute or two, until they blew the whistle to recommence play. And then, a wonderful idea popped into my head.

I took my place at the service line and served the ball in the exact same way. But this time, during the follow through, just as my right hand was about to nail me in the face once again, I simply reached up with my left hand and caught my right one, an inch or two in front of my face. I'm sure it looked silly, but it worked. My serves were an asset, not a liability, to our team.

That's cancer for you. You've got to roll with the punches. You've got to do your best to adjust to the new realities it brings, whatever they are.

For me, those realities have been devastating. While the first half of 2004 went rather well, things went downhill fast, and 2004 wound up being, by far, our worst year of all. Things became so bad that I will probably never be able to write about it. The painful memories are simply too much to face.

In August of 2004, we learned that cancer had returned to my arm, this time wrapping itself around my all-important nerve, which controlled the feeling in my hand. I was given the option of trying one more radical arm-saving surgery, but it was indeed a long-shot. "You're pretty much looking at an arm versus a life," one doctor said.

I had to make the terrifying call to have the doctors amputate my arm at the shoulder. And in so doing, I plunged into a darkness like no other, awaiting a scary, unknowable future that would test everything I had. The time leading to this surgery grew more painful and terrifying as each day passed, as I said goodbye to so many things that I'd never be able to do again, as I received one last call from a faith healer, begging me to forego surgery and try (that is, buy) some of his medicinal manna.

The last night was the grimmest of them all. LeAnn and I spent it alone in a Houston hotel, holding each other, and trying to find our way through.

The surgery took place on September 20, 2004. I was two months shy of my forty-first birthday.

Life on this side of surgery is completely different than it was before. Nearly everything has changed, and very little of that change has been good—but that's another book, *I Survived an Amputation, but Never Became the Bionic Man.*

The good news is that I've now been "cancer-free" for a year and a half. That's nearly twice as long as I'd ever made it before. The "cancer years," as I now call them, a five year period of trials and tribulations and some triumphs, are beginning to seem like a thing of the past. Let's hope so. For the sake of my friends and family, let's hope so.

In the end, the title to this book became strangely prophetic. I became that "things didn't turn out so great for him" guy I'd never wanted to be. But that's life my friends. And in a great many cases, that's cancer. We can't all wear the yellow jacket. Most of us are still in the peleton, struggling up the mountain.

FAVORITE

My doctor and I are buddies
even though she cut off my arm.

I've never had a friend lop off
one of my appendages before.
It's a little awkward at times,
disarticulating,
for we don't always know
what this means to our relationship.

She says I'm "one of her favorites."
But on some level that cannot be,
for I'm sure I bring her pain
just as she brings pain to me.

We share an unspoken bond—
a Lance Armstrong tale gone wrong.

Acknowledgments

Getting a book published is no easy task. If it were only a matter of writing and editing, that would be hard enough. For the process of conceptualizing and then actually writing an entire book is exceptionally difficult. There's a good reason so many dream of becoming writers, but never get beyond chapter one. It's a tough, lonely gig. And then, to write well…That's something else altogether.

But writing's only half the battle. The other half is to somehow sell your idea to others, which means working hard and becoming tough-skinned. There are many great writers out there who are never discovered, simply because they are horrible on the marketing end. There are many others who cannot stand the pain of criticism or, even worse, indifference.

To be honest, while attempting to get this book published, I had some moments of despair that rivaled some of my worst cancer experiences. Time after time, the book was "this close" to being a done deal, only to be followed by that crushing call, letter, or email. I did the whole "get yourself an agent" thing, only to find my year under contract with an agent frustrating and a waste of time. I've had sponsors firmly committed to the project suddenly pull out for unspoken reasons. One (formerly) dear friend read the book, found it too shocking for his Christian ears, and then shared that opinion with a would-be publisher.

In disheartening times like these, I found you've got to keep believing in yourself, or your book is dead in the water. Fortunately, I've had a lot of people who have believed in me and have been instrumental players in my publishing journey. Without their support, I never would have found my way.

During the writing process, Don Hull and John Storm (along with John's wife Susan) read and commented on my work in progress. Their thoughts and encouragement helped me to begin believing that the project was worthwhile.

Others read chapters of the book and provided constructive criticism and positive feedback. This list includes Lavonn Brown, Nathan Brown, Steffie Corcoran, R.C. Davis, Tom and Beverly Dowdy, Gary Fast, Marilyn Geiger, Tony Grider, Valerae Lewis, Jim Martin, and Lynn Weber. Their efforts on my behalf went above and beyond.

Others offered networking help. Brooks Hull was a tireless advocate on my behalf. Beth Cox, Lou Kohlman, Jana and Alan Moring, William and Ginger Murray, Dwight and Pam Normile, Jeanne Hoffman Smith, and Heather Poole all went to bat for me in one way or another, and I owe them all for those efforts.

I met with many writers/artists to discuss their experiences and seek their advice. Molly Griffis, Marcia Preston, Sandi Soli, Kathryn Jenson White, and Mike Wimmer come to mind. They each sat down with me at breakfast or lunch and listened to me blab.

Others who have supported me in important ways include Kirk Bjornsgaard, James Childress, Rob Collins, Billy Crockett, the Dream Institute, Carla Gildhouse, Linda McGuire, Jill Patterson, and the Sarcoma Alliance.

Please note that the poem "Tusks" appeared previously in *Blood and Thunder: Musings on the Art of Medicine*. The poem "Favorite" and other selections have been published in *The Blue Rock Review*.

Of course, this book would not have been possible without the vote of confidence from HAWK Publishing. This includes owner and novelist William Bernhardt and my fabulous editor, Jodie Nida, who has also authored many books. Oklahoma needs good people like this—people who are willing to go to bat for the little people and the little books they write. Hopefully their efforts and trust will be handsomely repaid when this book becomes an international bestseller. (Yes, I dream big!)

Thanks to Mom and Dad, Louise and Garold, Terry and Kathy, and the rest of my extended family. You've supported my family in so many ways during these horrible cancer years. It's been a team effort, and I thank you for all you've done.

And finally, thanks to my family, my inner circle, LeAnn, Maddye, and Ford. You've endured so much in the last several years, more than anyone could ever expect, but still you've stuck by me. Thank you for being there, for loving me despite my flaws and crazy ways, and for believing in me as husband, father, and writer. I love you all, and I'm so proud of who you are and what you do.